Care for the Liver Failure Patient

Editor

CYNTHIA C. BENZ

CRITICAL CARE NURSING CLINICS OF NORTH AMERICA

www.ccnursing.theclinics.com

Consulting Editor
DEBORAH GARBEE

September 2022 • Volume 34 • Number 3

ELSEVIER

1600 John F. Kennedy Boulevard • Suite 1800 • Philadelphia, Pennsylvania, 19103-2899

http://www.theclinics.com

CRITICAL CARE NURSING CLINICS OF NORTH AMERICA Volume 34, Number 3
September 2022 ISSN 0899-5885, ISBN-13: 978-0-323-98761-5

Editor: Kerry Holland
Developmental Editor: Ann Gielou M. Posedio

Critical Care Nursing Clinics of North America (ISSN 0899-5885) is published quarterly by Elsevier Inc., 360 Park Avenue South, New York, NY 10010-1710. Months of issue are March, June, September, and December. Business and Editorial Offices: 1600 John F. Kennedy Blvd., Suite 1800, Philadelphia, PA 19103-2899. Periodicals postage paid at New York, NY and additional mailing offices. Subscription prices are $160.00 per year for US individuals, $593.00 per year for US institutions, $100.00 per year for US students and residents, $206.00 per year for Canadian individuals, $611.00 per year for Canadian institutions, $230.00 per year for international individuals, $611.00 per year for international institutions, $115.00 per year for international students/residents and $100.00 per year for Canadian students/residents. To receive student/resident rate, orders must be accompanied by name of affiliated institution, data of term, and the *signature* of program/residency coordinator on institution letterhead. Orders will be billed at individual rate until proof of status is received. Foreign air speed delivery is included in all *Clinics* subscription prices. All prices are subject to change without notice. **POSTMASTER:** Send address changes to *Critical Care Nursing Clinics of North America*, Elsevier Health Sciences Division, Subscription Customer Service, 3251 Riverport Lane, Maryland Heights, MO 63043. **Customer Service: 1-800-654-2452 (US and Canada); 314-447-8871 (outside US and Canada). Fax: 314-447-8029. E-mail:** JournalsCustomerService-usa@elsevier.com **(for print support) and** JournalsOnlineSupport-usa@elsevier.com **(for online support).**

Reprints. For copies of 100 or more of articles in this publication, please contact the Commercial Reprints Department, Elsevier Inc., 360 Park Avenue South, New York, New York, 10010-1710; Tel.: 212-633-3874, Fax: 212-633-3820, and E-mail: reprints@elsevier.com.

Critical Care Nursing Clinics of North America is covered in *MEDLINE/PubMed (Index Medicus), International Nursing Index, Nursing Citation Index, Cumulative Index to Nursing and Allied Health Literature,* and *RNdex Top 100.*

Contributors

CONSULTING EDITOR

DEBORAH GARBEE, PhD, APRN, ACNS-BC, FCNS
Associate Dean for Professional Practice, Community Service and Advanced Nursing
Practice, Professor of Clinical Nursing, Louisiana State University Health Sciences Center
New Orleans School of Nursing, Louisiana, New Orleans

EDITOR

CYNTHIA C. BENZ, DNP, APRN
Clinical Nurse Specialist, Southeast Louisiana Veteran Health Care System, New Orleans,
Louisiana

AUTHORS

MARIE ADORNO, PhD, APRN, CNS, RNC-MNN, CNE
Director of the Nursing Research Doctorate Programs, Louisiana State University Health
New Orleans School of Nursing, New Orleans, Louisiana

LATANJA L. DIVENS, PhD, DNP, APRN, FNP-BC
Program Coordinator: Primary Care Adult-Gerontology and Family Nurse Practitioner
Programs, Assistant Professor of Clinical Nursing, Louisiana State University Health
New Orleans, School of Nursing, New Orleans, Louisiana

LOUISE FLYNN, MSN, RN
APRN, Solid Organ Transplant, Nemours Children's Hospital, Wilmington, Delaware

TONORA GARBUTT, DNP, RN, NEA-BC
Clinical Command Center Manager, Central Virginia Veterans Affairs Medical Center,
Richmond, Virginia

HOCHONG GILLES, DNP, FNP-BC, AF-AASLD
Clinical Program Director, Central Virginia Veterans Affairs Medical Center, Richmond,
Virginia

HEATHER ROSE GRUSH ABADIE, DNP, RNC-OB
Adjunct Faculty Herzing University, Metairie, Louisiana

CATHERINE HAUT, DNP, CPNP-AC/PC, CCRN, FAANP, FAAN
Director of Nursing Research and Evidence Based Practice, Nemours Children's Hospital,
Nursing Administration, Wilmington, Delaware; PICU Nurse Practitioner, Pediatrix Medical
Group, Baltimore, Maryland

JASMINE LANDRUM, DNP, RN
Endoscopy Nurse, Central Virginia Veterans Affairs Medical Center, Richmond, Virginia

NIKKI LEDOUX, BSN, RN
Transplant Coordinator, Southeast Louisiana Veterans Health Care System, New Orleans, Louisiana

CATHY MAHER-GRIFFITHS, DNS, RN, NEA-BC, RNC-OB
VP Quality Woman's Hospital, Baton Rouge, Louisiana

JILLIAN N. MAURIELLO, MSN, ARNP-C
Nurse Practitioner, Cardiology, Hunter Holmes McGuire VA Medical Center, Richmond, Virginia

CATHY McATEE, DNP, CCRN, ACNP-BC, CNE
Clinical Instructor, Adult Gerontology, Acute Care Nurse Practitioner Program, Louisiana Health Science Center New Orleans, New Orleans, Louisiana

HEATHER M. McCURDY, MSN
Nurse Practitioner, Gastroenterology Section, VA Ann Arbor Healthcare System, Ann Arbor, Michigan

ANNA M. NOBBE, MSN
Nurse Practitioner, Department of Digestive Diseases, Cincinnati VA Medical Center, Cincinnati, Ohio

VICKIE REED, DNP, APRN-NP, C
Hepatology Nurse Practitioner, Advanced Liver Disease Department, North-Western Iowa Veterans Administration Medical Center, Omaha, Nebraska

SHERRY L. RIVERA, DNP, APRN, ANP-C, FNKF
Assistant Professor of Clinical Nursing, Louisiana State University Health New Orleans, School of Nursing, Fellow of the National Kidney Foundation, New Orleans, Louisiana

MICHELLE M. STRAUGHAN, MSN, ARNP-C
Nurse Practitioner, Medicine, Gulf Coast Veterans Health Care System, Biloxi, Mississippi

JEANETTE VAUGHAN, DNP, RN, CCRN, CNL
Instructor of Nursing, Louisiana State University Health Sciences Center New Orleans, New Orleans, Louisiana

WHITNEY VILLEGAS, DNP, AGACNP-BC
Advanced Practice Provider, Trauma and Acute Care Emergency Surgery, John Peter Smith Health Network

QUENELL ZACHARIE DOUGLAS, MSN, APRN, FNP-C
Nurse Practitioner, Gastroenterology, Southeast Louisiana Veterans Health Care System, New Orleans, Louisiana

Contents

Pediatric acute liver failure is a rare diagnosis which can result in death or multiorgan system failure with a potential need for liver transplantation. The causative factors are many, but etiology, definitive pathophysiology, and directed therapies are still under investigation contributing to the difficulty in planning and providing both medical and nursing care. Clinical practice guidelines for acute liver failure are available for adult patients and through a national published position paper for pediatrics, but quality evidence is limited, especially with regard to testing and treatment recommendations, providing challenges in pediatric critical care decision making.

Hepatitis B can cause liver failure from both an acute infection and reactivation. Reactivation of hepatitis B has been associated with the use of direct-acting antivirals to treat hepatitis C and immunosuppressive therapies. This article discusses hepatitis B, acute liver failure, treatment, and supportive care. Liver transplantation is often the only option for patients with acute liver failure due to hepatitis B. Assessing for hepatitis B exposure and providing the hepatitis B vaccine will reduce the number of acute liver failure cases related to chronic hepatitis B.

Drug-induced liver injury (DILI) is a spectrum of liver injuries that can be classified by phenotype and injury patterns. Some injury patterns can be predicted in a number of drugs that are commonly used in practice, but idiosyncratic reactions are unpredictable and are not dose related. There are diagnostic criteria to assist in the classification of DILI phenotype as well as therapeutic interventions to ensure maximal support to the patient affected with DILI to include referral for liver transplantation in some cases.

Preeclampsia (PE) is the most common complication of pregnancy. PE is a multisystem disorder that can result in maternal morbidity and mortality. A severe complication of PE is the HELLP syndrome. HELLP syndrome is a pregnancy-associated liver disease characterized by the presence of hemolysis (H), elevated liver enzymes, and low platelet count. Management of HELLP syndrome includes monitoring of obstetric complications, controlling hypertension, seizure prevention, and planning for delivery. Also, postpartum care of the mother and the newborn should focus on physiologic and emotional wellbeing.

Hepatocellular carcinoma (HCC) is a primary liver malignancy commonly encountered in the setting of chronic liver disease and cirrhosis. Survival in HCC is determined by the ABCs: (A) anatomic stage; (B) biologic grade; and (C) cirrhosis severity. Improvement of imaging techniques permits clinicians to accurately diagnose HCC without biopsy confirmation. Advances in surgical and therapeutic options have improved treatment response and survival. Surgical resection, liver transplant, and thermal ablation in selected patients can potentially cure HCC. Noncurative approaches including intraarterial, radiation, and systemic therapies aim to palliate or slow the progression of disease. Management of HCC is complex, and the choice of treatment approach is enhanced by multidisciplinary consensus, including a liver transplant center.

Gastroesophageal variceal (GEV) bleeding is one of the most fatal complications of cirrhosis and can result in increased morbidity and mortality rates. This discussion focuses on management of acute gastrointestinal bleeding caused by esophageal and gastric varices and measures aimed at prevention of an initial or secondary GEV bleed.

Ascites is the most common and often the first decompensating event that occurs in cirrhosis. It has both a high symptom burden and high mortality rate. Increased abdominal girth, generalized abdominal pain, early satiety, and shortness of breath have a negative impact on quality of life. Treatments used to manage ascites include dietary sodium restriction, diuretics, large volume paracentesis, and transjugular intrahepatic portosystemic shunt. Secondary complications of ascites include refractory ascites, hyponatremia, and hepatorenal syndrome and are associated with reduced survival. Consideration should be given to the appropriateness and timing of referrals for liver transplant and/or palliative care.

Cirrhosis is a complex disease and has devastating effects on the liver. People living with the condition are at risk for many complications such as hepatorenal syndrome (HRS). If diagnosed with this condition, the prognosis is often poor. Therefore, it is imperative that treating providers are aware of the symptoms and methods to either prevent or adequately treat the syndrome. Timely referral, prevention, early recognition, and initiation of treatment are key components for prevention or improving the prognosis for HRS. Excluding potentially contributing factors and/or conditions is also vitally important for diagnostic purposes. Comorbid conditions may be present and further complicate diagnosis. Fluid volume replacement, administration of albumin, and vasoconstrictors as warranted are important for improving the hemodynamic status and potential reversal of HRS-acute kidney injury (HRS-AKI).

This article aims to focus on identifying hepatic encephalopathy (HE) due to portal hypertension and cirrhosis and implementing the most appropriate treatment. The occurrence of hepatic encephalopathy is prognostic in the life expectancy and quality of life of individuals with cirrhosis. Patients diagnosed with cirrhosis should be thoroughly assessed for HE. Many studies have identified that even HE in a subclinical (covert) presentation is a predicator of increased mortality before and after liver transplant. HE, rather minimal or overt, indicates diminished quality of life, increased health care dollars and mortality.

Currently, there are 6.2 million people with heart failure (HF) in the United States with 1 million new HF cases being diagnosed annually. Twenty to 30% of patients with acute heart failure also have liver dysfunction. The dual diagnoses of chronic heart and liver disease has significant prognostic implications.

The liver is the most frequently damaged organ in abdominal trauma. There is a high risk of hemorrhage and mortality as severity of injury and stage increases. During the last decade, management of liver trauma standards changed when the American Association of the Surgery of Trauma adjusted their guidelines to focus on early computed tomography scanning to determine the severity of liver injury trauma and the need for surgical verses nonsurgical management. Liver injury can be blunt or penetrating. Trauma teams became more multidisciplinary to focus not only on the physical but also on the psychosocial issues with trauma. Algorithms were developed to guide trauma flow and determination of severity of injury by grade. Nursing considerations and management include maintaining hemodynamic stability via accurate fluid resuscitation, monitoring of frequent vitals signs and abdominal assessment. Care must be taken to address pain and the psychosocial and emotional issues of trauma.

CRITICAL CARE NURSING CLINICS OF NORTH AMERICA

SERIES OF RELATED INTEREST

Nursing Clinics of North America http://www.nursing.theclinics.com

THE CLINICS ARE AVAILABLE ONLINE!
Access your subscription at:
www.theclinics.com

In Memoriam

Latanja Divens, PhD, DNP, APRN, FNP-BC (1974-2022)

Every day is a gift

—Dr Latanja Divens

Dr Latanja L. Divens, an Assistant Professor of Clinical Nursing and the Program Coordinator for the BSN to DNP Adult Gerontology Primary Care and Family Nurse Practitioner Programs at the Louisiana State University Health New Orleans School of Nursing, touched the hearts and lives of everyone she encountered. She is survived by her devoted husband, Kiel Divens, and her loving family.

She challenged herself and those around her to achieve their highest potential. She obtained a Bachelor of Science from Xavier University, a Bachelor of Science from Holy Cross College, a Master of Science, and a Doctor of Nursing Practice from Loyola University. As a Nurse Practitioner, she was passionate about providing high-quality primary care and a desire to help others. She especially enjoyed providing care to patients with chronic diseases. In 2018, she achieved a Doctor of Philosophy from William Carey University. Her doctoral thesis was about the professional development and practice readiness of Family Nurse Practitioner students.

She was affectionately known as Dr Dr Divens to those of us who knew and loved her. As a Registered Nurse, Nurse Practitioner, and Nurse Educator, she inspired countless nurses and nurse practitioners to provide compassionate, high-quality care to the patients that they serve.

Crit Care Nurs Clin N Am 34 (2022) ix
https://doi.org/10.1016/j.cnc.2022.05.001
0899-5885/22/© 2022 Published by Elsevier Inc.

Preface

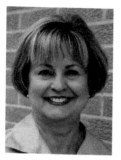

Cynthia C. Benz, DNP, APRN
Editor

Patients with liver failure present many challenges for health care providers. The liver performs a multitude of physiologic functions that maintain the normal homeostasis of the body. The liver processes protein, detoxifies drugs and toxins, regulates glucose, and synthesizes coagulation factors to facilitate homeostasis. When these functions are stressed, health care providers are confronted with challenges caring for the seriously ill patient with liver disease. This issue of *Critical Care Nursing Clinics of North America* focuses on a few of the causes of acute liver failure (ALF) and common complications associated with both acute and chronic liver failure.

ALF is a sudden onset of liver injury often considered a life-threatening event and is accompanied by coagulopathy and encephalopathy. Several causes of ALF are discussed in great detail in this issue: acute hepatitis B, drug-induced liver failure, pediatric liver trauma, and the HELLP syndrome. Early recognition and management of these complex conditions are essential for the survival of the patient.

Cirrhosis is the last stage of fibrosis development and is often asymptomatic. Cirrhosis is often associated with multiple complications. Some of those complications are discussed in this issue: hepatocellular carcinoma, bleeding esophageal varices, spontaneous bacterial peritonitis, and hepatorenal syndrome. Each of these complications can be life threatening. Once again, prompt recognition and management of these complications are critical to achieve positive patient care outcomes.

Cynthia C. Benz, DNP, APRN
Southeast Louisiana Veteran Health Care System
2400 Canal Street
New Orleans, LA 70119, USA

E-mail address:
Cynthia.Benz@va.gov

Crit Care Nurs Clin N Am 34 (2022) xi
https://doi.org/10.1016/j.cnc.2022.04.001
0899-5885/22/© 2022 Published by Elsevier Inc.

Acute Liver Failure in Children

Catherine Haut, DNP, CPNP-AC/PC, CCRN[a,b,*], Louise Flynn, MSN, RN[c,d]

KEYWORDS

- Pediatric liver failure • Liver failure • Pediatric acute liver failure

KEY POINTS

- Pediatric acute liver failure is extremely rare but rapidly progressive with significant morbidity and mortality.
- Evidence regarding diagnostic testing and definitive diagnosis, pathophysiology, and directed treatment is limited in the literature.
- Nurses caring for pediatric patients in the critical care setting need to be aware of the conditions that can contribute to the development of acute liver failure.
- Critical care management of children with acute liver failure is aimed at preventing, identifying, and rapidly addressing multisystem organ failure.

INTRODUCTORY CASE STUDY

A previously healthy 5-year-old child arrives at the emergency department comatose with unknown etiology. The child is determined to be in fulminant liver failure with elevation of liver enzymes and hyperammonemia and is emergently admitted to the pediatric intensive care unit (PICU). She has no known history of liver disease but recently had a viral illness. She rapidly develops multisystem organ failure and requires invasive ventilation, fluid resuscitation, and inotropic therapy. The child remains in liver failure, so high-volume plasmapheresis (HVP) is initiated and planning for emergent liver transplant is begun. The child's eligibility for transplant and prognosis for recovery remain questionable. Family members are distraught and health care providers have difficulty understanding the mechanisms surrounding this rapid deterioration.

[a] Nemours Children's Hospital, Nursing Administration, 1600 Rockland Road, Wilmington, DE 19803, USA; [b] Pediatrix Medical Group, Baltimore, MD, USA; [c] APRN, Solid Organ Transplant, Nemours Children's Hospital, Wilmington, DE, USA; [d] Department, Solid Organ Transplant, Nemours Children's Health, 1600 Rockland Road, Wilmington, DE 19803, USA
* Corresponding author. Nemours Children's Hospital, Delaware, 1600 Rockland Road, Wilmington, DE 19803.
E-mail address: Catherine.haut@nemours.org

Crit Care Nurs Clin N Am 34 (2022) 241–258
https://doi.org/10.1016/j.cnc.2022.04.002
0899-5885/22/© 2022 Elsevier Inc. All rights reserved.
ccnursing.theclinics.com

Abbreviations	
PT	prothrombin time
OT	occupational Therapy
AST	aspartate Aminotransferase
ALT	alanine Aminotransferase
ROM	range of Motion
NPO	nothing by Mouth
EBNA	epstein-Barr Virus Nuclear Antigen
IGG	immunoglobulin G
IGM	immunoglobulin M
CT	computerized Tomography
EEG	electroencephalogram
CBC	complete Blood Count
ANA	antinuclear Antibodies
ANCA	antineutrophil Cytoplasmic Anibodies
SMA	smooth Muscle Antibody
LKMA	anti-Liver-KidneyMicrosome Antibody
IL	interleukin CD25 Interleukin-2-receptor alpha chain
NSS	normal Saline Solution
HP	haptoglobin
BP	blood Pressure
NG	nasogastric

BACKGROUND

Pediatric acute liver failure (PALF) is rare, often occurring in previously healthy children for varied reasons, but up to 40% of the time etiology is unknown.[1,2] Children with acute liver failure (ALF) can have rapidly progressive illness, develop multisystem organ failure and approximately 30% will require transplantation or die. However, owing to the nature of "young" organs and the process of regeneration, some of these patients will experience a full recovery with return of liver function. PALF or pediatric fulminant liver failure is a syndrome managed in the ICU, and therapies are often based on center preferences due to a lack of quality evidence and research conducted with large sample size.

In the United States, the death rate from ALF in all populations is approximately 13.5 per 100,000 population annually.[3] An estimated 500 to 600 children are diagnosed with ALF annually in the United States, but the actual number of children who die from ALF is unknown.[4] Unfortunately, it is difficult to identify those children who will be significantly affected by PALF and to make decisions for transplant when patient status is critical. Organ procurement and transplant are also processes that require experience and expertise, not readily available in every pediatric hospital. Ultimately children with ALF require pediatric critical care services in a location with a liver transplant team available.

DEFINITION/HISTORY

A better understanding of PALF begins with an acceptable, comprehensive definition that has historically been hard to specify and documented to be ambiguous. There are several published statements that can define or explain the phenomena, which include biochemical evidence of liver injury in children without chronic liver disease; coagulopathy not corrected with vitamin K administration, and international normalized ratio

(INR) of greater than 1.5 in a child with encephalopathy or greater than 2.0 in a child without encephalopathy.[4,5] The original definition of PALF was derived from the adult definition of severe ALF for fewer than 26 weeks duration with evidence of hepatic encephalitis (HE) and INR of 1.5 or higher in a patient without preexisting liver disease or cirrhosis.[6] Children do not always present with encephalitis, and symptoms and findings are different and etiology and treatment are not parallel compared with that for adults. Children with chronic liver failure, such as that encountered with biliary atresia (BA) can present with acute-on chronic liver failure (ACLF) and will also require critical care management with potential for urgent transplantation.

Historical perspectives of PALF begin in the early 1600s, with documentation of children who had fever, jaundice, and neurologic dysfunction and then in the 1800s with same symptoms and use of the description "acute yellow atrophy."[4] In the mid-1900s, scientists began to associate certain pharmaceuticals and hepatitis with ALF and in 1953, a large study of patients who had died from ALF explained some rationale for liver failure in seven children to include exposure to halothane, infectious or serum hepatitis, and Reye syndrome.[4] In 1980, single-center retrospective reports of ALF in children emerged, followed by a large multicenter study that included 348 children, describing the etiology and clinical findings including HE and 3-week outcomes.[7] Correlates within this study indicate that encephalopathy was not an absolute requirement for diagnosis, almost half of these children did not have a specific diagnosis and the causes of PALF were different than in adults. Outcomes and diagnosis between younger age groups (age < 1 year) and those in ages ranging up to 18 years were also differentiated.[7]

The history of liver transplant is also of interest when considering PALF. Before 1970, most children with ALF died. The first liver transplant in the United States took place in 1963, but attempts continued to be unsuccessful until 1967, when a 1 ½-year-old child was transplanted for liver carcinoma and lived 13 months, passing away from metastasis.[8] Successful transplants continued and today, the long-term survival rates in children can be greater than 85%.[8,9]

Etiology

Liver failure in the pediatric patient can result from a variety of factors representing both acute and chronic illnesses. Congenital reasons for liver failure occurring in infancy include BA and metabolic disorders, but infectious diseases account for the majority of cases in infancy.[5] The most common reason for liver transplant in children is BA, which is typically considered a chronic illness, occurring in 6.5 to 7.5 infants per 100,000 live births in the United States and can be congenital or acquired in which infants are normal appearing at birth and develop symptoms weeks or months later.[10,11] BA involves the obstruction of extra-hepatic bile ducts resulting in the obstruction of bile flow out of the liver. Acquired BA or undiagnosed illness can result in PALF, so it is important to include this illness when discussing ALF.[4]

Most acute events in children resulting in ALF include toxic ingestion, primarily from medications, infectious or viral illness, shock from infection or other entity, status epilepticus, and trauma. Intentional overdose or accidental ingestion of acetaminophen is one of the most common presentations of PALF.[2] Primary causes of PALF are different whether occurring in the United States or other countries.[2] In developing countries where hepatitis A vaccine is not required, and in countries where hepatitis A is endemic, the incidence of PALF is higher than in developed countries where the vaccine is part of preventive care, as the United States.[12] A systematic review of 32 articles representing 18 countries identified acetaminophen toxicity as the main cause of PALF in developed countries, followed by metabolic disorders and infection, with almost 40% of cases with indeterminable cause.[1] For infants under the age of 1 residing in developing countries, unspecified infection was the highest causative factor followed by metabolic disease and then cytomegalovirus (CMV) infection.[1] In the United States, the etiology of PALF is classified as infectious, immunologic, metabolic, and toxin/drug related.[13] Viral infections can include CMV, Epstein–Barr virus (EBV), enterovirus, adenovirus and herpes simplex virus. Immunologic causes of PALF include autoimmune hepatitis (AIH), sclerosing cholangitis, and AIH following liver transplant.[13]

Metabolic diseases contributing to the development of PALF include galactosemia, tyrosinemia, urea cycle defects, and fatty acid oxidation disorders, among others, with those occurring in neonates identified through newborn screening.[5] Wilson disease is a hereditary metabolic disorder, described as a gene mutation with progressive illness characterized by the accumulation of toxic levels of copper in the liver, brain, and other organs, including the corneas of the eyes, neurologic system, kidneys, and heart. Kayser–Fleischer rings are found with copper deposition in the corneas and patients can exhibit neurologic changes as initial symptoms. Wilson disease is typically diagnosed over the age of 5 years and is fatal without treatment. However, most children with Wilson disease do not require transplantation.[14,15]

Drug toxicity, primarily acetaminophen, is a common cause of PALF but has an excellent prognosis if treated emergently based on the time of ingestion and if HE is not present.[13] Other medications responsible for PALF, include those classified as antiepileptic, anti-infective, including quinolones and macrolides, immunomodulatory, and anti-inflammatory agents, along with herbal and dietary supplements and recreational drugs such as cocaine and mushrooms.[13] PALF can also be associated with multisystem response to illness or injury contributing to hypoperfusion to the liver, which includes shock, hypotension, vaso-occlusive disease, and trauma. Oncologic diagnoses, such as hepatoblastoma and inflammatory syndromes, can also affect liver function.

With the advent of COVID-19, there are case studies and small sample retrospective reviews identifying ALF not only in hospitalized adult patients but also in children diagnosed with acute COVID-19 infection and multisystem inflammatory syndrome.[16] It has been noted that 14% to 53% of all patients admitted to the hospital with a primary diagnosis of COVID-19 had elevated liver transaminases.[16] Pathology suggests that hepatocellular infection or an inflammatory or autoimmune response from COVID-19 can lead to PALF and hepatic steatosis.[17,18] Patients with underlying liver abnormalities, including cirrhosis or chronic liver disease, have an increased likelihood of morbidity and mortality from COVID-19 and patients who had transplants were at higher risk of severe disease based on the use of immunotherapy post transplant.[16]

Finally, PALF can be incidental, when children present with neurologic/psychological abnormalities and elevated liver enzymes including bilirubin level.

PATHOPHYSIOLOGY

The three primary functions of the liver include synthesis, detoxification, and excretion, but the liver is responsible for many processes. Production of proteins with the regulation of blood levels of amino acids, conversion of glucose into glycogen, blood clotting, and iron storage are just a few of these functions. As blood passes through the liver, it is responsible for breaking down, balancing and creating nutrients, metabolizing drugs and other substances, and excretion of bile that assists in carrying waste products.[13] The liver has immune properties, which are important for infection resistance and removing bacteria from the blood. Cellular components such as hepatocytes, epithelial cells, lymphocytes, and T cells are involved in the immune response when an infectious substance is introduced. Liver injury is associated with an inflammatory or autoimmune response with abrupt hepatocyte injury.[13] Acute insult to the liver can cause loss of synthetic function, which is marked by abnormal values of albumin, bilirubin, and prothrombin time, with associated thrombosis or hypercoagulability versus concern for bleeding.[19] The liver is mostly an efficient organ in which injury or insult from toxins can result in a brief increase in serum aminotransferases/enzymes versus fulminant liver failure. However, just as the etiology of PALF is often unknown, the pathology related to a specific diagnosis or rationale for PALF may be unknown or not understood.

Children with chronic liver disease or failure can have acute events, resulting in hospitalization and PICU admission. As the liver is responsible for glucose, lipid, glucagon, and some hormone metabolism, chronic changes with liver fibrosis and cirrhosis result in insulin resistance and an increased potential for adrenal insufficiency.[20] Children who present with ACLF have a higher risk of mortality based on these underlying problems.[20]

PRESENTATION OF ACUTE DISEASE

Children with ALF present with varied symptoms and physical findings depending on age, acuity of illness and etiology. Physical findings of children with suspected chronic liver disease include failure to grow/thrive, hepatosplenomegaly, clubbing of fingers and toes, peripheral edema, and spider angiomas on the skin.[20] Acute presentation can include abnormal neurologic or psychological symptoms, fatigue, malaise, nausea and abdominal pain, fever, and jaundice.[21] It is important to elicit a thorough history, especially of ill contacts, recent travel, medications, and family history of metabolic illness or autoimmune disease, as well as considering any of the diagnoses that include acute liver insult. Abnormal laboratory results can be the first indication of suspected PALF or a child can present with fulminant liver failure, progressing to multisystem organ failure.[1]

Laboratory findings in PALF include coagulation abnormalities with elevated INR and prolonged PT, low platelet count, and decreased fibrinogen. Elevated transaminases, including AST and ALT, and hyperammonemia with hypoglycemia, hyponatremia and other electrolyte abnormalities or acid-base disturbances.

Diagnosis and Recommended Studies

Clinical practice guidelines of the American Gastroenterological Association Institute have been published with recommendations intended for adult patients, representing similar treatments for children, but due to the limited research opportunity with large sample sizes, the evidence is not strong with support for many therapies.[22] A position paper published by the North American Society of Pediatric Gastroenterology, Hepatology and Nutrition, updated in January 2022, provides PALF historical information, recommendations for diagnostic testing, referral, and imaging.[4] **Table 1** shows the suggested age-based approaches for laboratory studies, imaging, and other procedures, such as liver biopsy, based on national recommendations that were collated by this hospital's solid organ transplant team. Common diagnostic testing for Wilson disease is included with this list; serum ceruloplasmin, serum and hepatic copper levels, and a 24-h urine collection for copper, but may not be reliable for the definitive documentation of Wilson disease. Regardless, the extent of testing is important in assisting the identification of potential causative factors, which can guide treatment.[14] Obtaining laboratory studies to assess coagulation status, oxygen-carrying capacity as

Table 1
Pediatric acute liver failure recommended work-up

	Age Group < 3 mo	Ages 3 mo to 18 y
Priority Testing: Infectious Etiology	Enterovirus blood Polymerase chain reaction (PCR)* Adenovirus blood PCR* Influenza A and B rapid (seasonal)* *Rapid viral panel can be done to test for all Cytomegalovirus (CMV) blood PCR, IGG, IGM Epstein Barr virus (EBV) panel IGM, IGG, EBNA Hepatitis A IGM/IGG Hepatitis B sAg, sAb core Ag, blood PCR Hepatitis C sAb, blood PCR Human Immunodeficiency Virus (HIV) blood PCR HIV 4th-generation testing Human herpes virus (HHV-6) blood PCR COVID-19 PCR Blood culture Parvovirus B19 PCR, IGM, IGG	Enterovirus blood PCR* Adenovirus blood PCR* Influenza A and B rapid (seasonal)* *Rapid viral panel can be done to test for all CMV blood PCR, IGG, IGM EBV panel IGM, IGG, EBNA Hepatitis A IGM/IGG Hepatitis B sAg, sAb core Ag, blood PCR Hepatitis C sAb, blood PCR HIV blood PCR HIV 4th-generation testing HHV-6 blood PCR COVID-19 PCR Blood culture Parvovirus B19 PCR, IGM, IGG
Consults/Referrals	Gastroenterology/ hepatology Intensive care Neurology Neurosurgery Nephrology Metabolic disease specialists Solid organ transplant surgeons *Consider social worker, dietician	Gastroenterology/ hepatology Intensive care Neurology Neurosurgery Nephrology Metabolic disease specialists Solid organ transplant surgeons *Consider social worker, dietician
Priority Non-Infectious Work-Up	Genetic testing* CBC with differential Complete metabolic panel Liver function tests Ferritin Serum amino acids Ammonia Lactate Pyruvate L/P ratio Plasma acylcarnitine profile Urine-reducing substances Urine succinylacetone Urine organic acids	Genetic testing* CBC with differential Complete metabolic panel Liver function tests Acetaminophen level Urine toxicology screen ANA, ANCA, SMA, LKMA, anti-F-actin Ab Total IGG with subtypes Lipid panel with triglyceride Ferritin, Fibrinogen, soluble IL2-R alpha (sCD25) Ceruloplasmin (4–18 y) Serum and hepatic copper

(continued on next page)

Table 1 (continued)		
	Age Group < 3 mo	**Ages 3 mo to 18 y**
	Urine orotic acid	24-h urine copper
	*based on individual case	Serum amino acids
		Ammonia
		Lactate
		Pyruvate
		L/P ratio
		Plasma acylcarnitine profile
		Urine organic acids
		*based on individual case
Imaging	MRI of abdomen and brain	Abdominal US w/Doppler
	Abdominal US w/Doppler	Abdominal CT
	Abdominal CT	Echocardiogram
	Echocardiogram	EEG*
	EEG*	*based on neurologic
	*based on neurologic	status and findings
	status and findings	
Procedures	Liver biopsy—per	Liver biopsy—per
	hepatology	hepatology
	*to include specific staining	*to include specific staining
	request (PALF-consistent	request (PALF-consistent
	lymphocytes)	lymphocytes)
	Buccal biopsy of minor	
	salivary glands	

* indicates that suggested testing, etc, may be individualized.
Table contents courtesy of Dr. Adebowale Adeyemi and Nemours Children's Hospital, Delaware
Solid Organ Transplant Team

reflected by hemoglobin and hematocrit, and electrolytes are the initial tasks for testing, followed by the determination of need for imaging studies and liver biopsy.

In addition to recommendations for diagnostic testing and referrals, review of the history and family history is important in determining the etiology of PALF. History questions include review of past diagnosis of liver failure or disease in other family members, previous infant death, exposure to recent illness, including COVID-19, previous blood transfusions, and known autoimmune conditions.[23] The onset of symptoms and family notation of mental status, skin color changes, or other physical findings are also important to document.

Critical Care Management and Potential Complications

Patients admitted to the PICU with PALF will require team-based care, involving specialty services beginning on admission with a comprehensive management plan for longer term goals. **Table 2** includes potential system-based complications and recommendations for treatment, which can be all encompassing, reflecting every body system. Encephalitis with cerebral edema is related to hyperammonemia, inflammatory response of illness, and increased cerebral blood flow and requires immediate attention.[23] Respiratory distress and failure can result from the underlying cause of PALF, but respiratory support would also be necessary if the child's neurologic status deteriorates. Peripheral vasodilation with intravascular volume depletion will present as hypotension and tachycardia, requiring fluid resuscitation and vasoconstrictive pharmacologic therapy.[23] There are multiple reasons for renal failure as another major

Table 2
Pediatric acute liver failure: System-based complications and management of complications

System	Potential Problems	Recommended Therapy/ Support
Neurologic *Encephalopathy Cerebral edema	Altered mental status Malaise, fatigue Seizures Coma	Continuous assessment Avoid stimulation or painful interventions Management of increased intracranial pressure with Mannitol, 3% saline Avoid hyponatremic states Decreasing Glasgow coma score (GCS): Intubation and ventilation
Respiratory	Respiratory distress and failure Acute respiratory distress syndrome Pulmonary hemorrhage	Ventilatory support Oxygenation Monitoring of oxygen saturation and end-tidal CO_2 Careful choices for sedation medications while monitoring neurologic status
Cardiac	Hypotension Tachycardia	Fluid resuscitation Use of inotropes/ vasoconstrictors if necessary (Norepinephrine)
Gastrointestinal/Nutrition	Gastrointestinal bleeding	H2 blockers or proton pump inhibitor for prophylaxis Enteral feedings with high calorie-dense formula
*Renal Fluid and Electrolytes	Acute kidney injury with renal failure Intravascular volume depletion Dehydration Altered electrolytes to include hypoglycemia and hyperammonemia Acidosis and alkalosis	Strict intake and output Fluid resuscitation with NSS, avoid free water Replacement of electrolytes and frequent monitoring Continuous renal-replacement therapy
Hematologic	Bleeding/coagulopathy not corrected with vitamin K administration Disseminated intravascular coagulation	Vitamin K administration Blood products if indicated/ caution for fluid overload
Infectious Disease	Viral infection Bacterial infection of any system Systemic inflammatory response syndrome	Monitor for fever Rapid viral panel testing COVID-19 testing Blood, urine cultures Appropriate antibiotic therapy

(continued on next page)

Table 2		
(continued)		
System	Potential Problems	Recommended Therapy/ Support
Psychosocial and Family Support		Explanations of all complications and therapy Encourage caregiver presence at bedside and comfort techniques

* indicates that suggested testing, etc, may be individualized.
Data from Tissieres P, Devictor DJ. Acute liver failure and liver transplantation. In Morrison W, Nelson McMillan KL, Shaffner D. *Rogers Handbook of Pediatric Intensive Care*, 5th edition. 2017: chapter 80:550-554. Wolters Kluwer, and Grek A, Arasi L. Acute liver failure. *AACNACConline.org.* 2016;27(4):420-429.

complication of PALF, including acetaminophen toxicity, nephrotoxic medications, hypovolemia, and sepsis. Monitoring kidney function and fluid and electrolyte status, primarily creatinine and urine output assist in determining treatment with continuous renal replacement therapy (CRRT). As the liver is involved in immune response, new infections can occur, requiring rapid identification and treatment. Decreased liver function results in coagulopathy, including low platelet count and increased INR, indicating the need for vitamin K and blood product administration. However, caution in the use of blood products is recommended, based on the possibility of fluid overload.

For children who are admitted with acute-on chronic liver failure, underlying cirrhosis and liver fibrosis complicate the course with an even higher mortality rate than PALF.[21] ACLF is associated with acute adrenal insufficiency requiring corticosteroid therapy and potential hyperglycemia with the need for insulin or an insulin drip for regulation as patients with cirrhosis can be insulin resistant. Additionally, this presentation can result in peripheral vasodilation with low systemic vascular resistance, with potential for hypotension and poor cardiac output.[20]

Children with ALF in the PICU may require intubation and ventilation, CRRT, and HVP, a technique for treatment of ALF while awaiting liver transplant. Typically, CRRT in PALF is treatment of renal failure and to remove circulating fluid volume but in some places has been adapted to address removal of toxins. There are systems that can be used for HVP, which include the use of fresh frozen plasma in the circuit to remove ammonia, circulating cytokines, protein-bound toxins, and other substances.[24,25] Therapy is intermittent and has been safe in children without procedure-related complications.[24,25]

Liver Transplant

There are approximately 500 liver transplants completed in children in the United States each year, with BA as the primary indication for the age group less than 2 years and nonalcoholic fatty liver disease increasing the transplant numbers in the adolescent age group.[26] Additional indications for liver transplant include alpha-1 antitrypsin deficiency, Alagille syndrome, cryptogenic cirrhosis, and autoimmune hepatitis.[9] The Children's Oncology Group recommends referral to a transplant program for children diagnosed with hepatoblastoma depending on pretreatment extent of disease stage.[27] Contraindications for liver transplant in children, including those with PALF are irreversible brain injury, ongoing infection, underlying cancer diagnosis, severe metabolic illness, or progressing cardiopulmonary disease or failure.[23] Children with ALF, represent about 10% of all liver transplants each year.[23]

The rejection rate is higher in patients who are acutely ill before transplant, so stabilization and support prior to the surgical procedure is important. Use of a model for end-stage liver disease (MELD) score for patients over the age of 12 or a pediatric end stage liver disease (PELD) score for those under age 12, can assist in determining the severity of liver disease or the estimated 90-day probability of death before the transplant.[28,29] The Organ Procurement and Transplantation Network utilizes this score to prioritize allocation of organs, targeting those who have higher scores.[30] The MELD score is based on biologic markers of liver function including lab values of INR, creatinine, bilirubin and sodium, and frequency of dialysis or CRRT. The PELD score uses albumin, bilirubin levels, and INR along with growth failure, based on height and weight measurements.[28,29] Controversy exists about MELD and PELD scores representing true need and urgency for organ donation.[29] An additional measurement is the status of pediatric patients for transplant purposes as labeled 1A and 1B. Status 1A patients have ALF and may not survive more than days without a transplant. Status 1B is a label specific to pediatric patients and identifies patients with specified chronic illness who are younger than 18 years of age.[30]

Nursing Care

Nursing care of patients with PALF should be system based and involves continuous monitoring, identification of hemodynamic instability, and acute altered neurologic status as priorities. Head-to-toe assessment includes monitoring neurologic status for HE and resultant cerebral edema, often difficult to accomplish effectively in young children. Cardiac evaluation includes frequent checks of heart rate, blood pressure, and peripheral perfusion, along with careful measurement of intake and output, reflective of fluid status and potential renal failure.[31] Vasodilation and hypotension are common findings in patients with sepsis, trauma, and ALF, occurring as effects of circulating cytokines and endotoxins.[31] Poor intake prior to admission can contribute to hypovolemia presenting as hypotension and tachycardia. Respiratory compromise can occur as a result of critical illness and altered neurologic status. Airway protection is essential, so management of ventilation and oxygenation is another nursing chore. Expect and support early nutrition, either enterally or parenterally along with frequent lab analysis. **Table 3** outlines directed nursing care for patients with PALF, those with ACLF and post transplant.

Other Considerations and Family Education

Including specialists in the care of children with PALF early in the illness trajectory is extremely important with inclusion of dieticians and social workers or case managers. Nutritional assessment and support are necessary in the PICU and before liver transplant. Children with ALF often have metabolic disorders and may present in a catabolic state. Enteral tube feeding and parenteral nutrition may be needed as nutrition can improve liver transplant outcomes. Nutrition is based on resting energy expenditure which is increased in ALF.[32]

Parents of children in the PICU experience stress and anxiety and feel loss of control, especially with an unexpected critical illness.[33] Multiple challenges for families exist that encompass emotional, spiritual, financial, and physical burdens especially as related to complex health care needs with uncertain outcomes. Caregivers who have children who need to undergo liver transplantation have increased daily responsibilities, including the provision of immunosuppressive therapy and worry about the risk of infection and overall financial burden, potentially lasting a lifetime. Research by Yahan and Duken (2019) indicates that parents of children post liver transplant cannot do social things, neglect housework, feel a sense of hopelessness, and

Table 3
Nursing care for the pediatric patient with acute liver failure, acute-on chronic liver failure and post-operative liver transplant

	Critical Care Considerations	Nursing Care Recommendations
Acute liver failure	Acute presentation: * Consider possible causes of presentation from history 1. Neurologic 2. Cardiovascular 3. Respiratory 4. Gastrointestinal/Metabolic 5. Muscular Skeletal/Integumentary 6. Infectious disease 7. Psychosocial	1. Complete nursing physical assessment/Neurologic evaluation • Vital signs • Neurologic status focus: GCS • Measure height and weight on admission 2. Frequent monitoring of HR, BP, and circulatory status • Fluid resuscitation • Vasoconstrictors/Inotropic medications as needed 3. Respiratory support and airway protection • Continuous pulse oximetry and respiratory assessment • Oxygen if indicated • Invasive or noninvasive ventilation if indicated • Intubation and ventilation for airway protection based on neurologic status 4. Fluid and electrolyte management/nutrition • Frequent monitoring of electrolytes with renal function, ammonia, and liver function tests • Resuscitation with isotonic fluids • Avoid/treat hyponatremia • Initial NPO status, enteral feeds when possible • Consider stomach protection with H2 blocker or proton pump inhibitor for stomach protection when NPO • Dietician consult for nutritional assessment, calories, and inclusion of specific nutrients • IV fluids, parenteral or enteral feedings based on patient status • Strict intake and output regimen • Ongoing weight measurement 5. Range of motion/Prevention of skin pressure areas/breakdown • Assessment and positioning • Consult PT/OT

(continued on next page)

Table 3 (continued)		
	Critical Care Considerations	**Nursing Care Recommendations**
		6. Consider possible causes of acute presentation to include viral or bacterial infection • Antibiotics for prophylaxis may be needed • CBC with differential and blood cultures • Other cultures as indicated 7. Patient and family support • Include family members/care providers in discussion of status and planning of care • Encourage family participation in caring for child and presence at bedside when possible • Consult social worker/case manager for counseling and support • Refer to transplant counselor if transplant is imminent
Acute on Chronic Liver Failure	Acute presentation: *Consider possible causes of presentation from history and physical findings 1. Neurologic 2. Cardiovascular 3. Respiratory 4. Gastrointestinal/metabolic: fluid and electrolytes 5. Muscular skeletal/ integumentary 6. Infectious disease 7. Psychosocial	1. Nursing physical assessment/ neurologic evaluation • Vital signs • Neurologic status focus: GCS • Signs of chronic state: ascites, failure to thrive • Measure height and weight on admission 2. Frequent monitoring of HR, BP, and circulatory status • Fluid resuscitation • Vasoconstrictors/inotropic medications 3. Respiratory support and airway protection • Evaluation of chronic status and previous respiratory support • Continuous pulse oximetry and respiratory assessment • Oxygen if indicated • Invasive or noninvasive ventilation if indicated • Intubation and ventilation for airway protection based on neurologic status 4. Fluid and electrolyte management/nutrition • Frequent monitoring of electrolytes with renal

(continued on next page)

Table 3
(continued)

Critical Care Considerations	Nursing Care Recommendations
	function, ammonia, and liver function tests
	• Resuscitation with isotonic fluids
	• Avoid/treat hyponatremia
	• Initial NPO status, enteral feeds when possible
	• Early nutritional assessment by dietician, awareness of diet regimen for chronic illness, and inclusion of needed nutrients
	• Consider stomach protection with H2 blocker or proton pump inhibitor for stomach protection when NPO
	• IV fluids, parenteral or enteral feedings based on patient status
	• Strict intake and output regimen
	• Ongoing weight measurement
	5. Assess previous ambulatory status/skin status
	• Assessment and positioning
	• Consult PT/OT as needed for ROM
	6. Consider possible causes of acute presentation to include viral or bacterial infection
	• Antibiotics for prophylaxis may be needed
	• If previous transplant, continue immunosuppressant medications
	• CBC with differential and blood cultures
	• Other cultures as indicated
	7. Involve parents/caregivers with plan of care
	• Consult social worker/case manager or those providing support for chronic illness in past
	• Include family members/care providers in discussion of status and planning of care
	• Encourage family participation in caring for child and presence at bedside when possible
	• Consider mental health evaluation and counseling for patient and family.

(continued on next page)

Table 3 (continued)		
	Critical Care Considerations	**Nursing Care Recommendations**
Post-Transplant Nursing Care	Post-Operative care: *After airway, breathing, and circulation, most important nursing care post transplant is support of organ function and recognition of possible graft dysfunction 1. Neurologic 2. Cardiovascular 3. Respiratory 4. Gastrointestinal 5. Metabolic: fluid and electrolytes 6. Muscular skeletal/ integumentary 7. Infectious disease 8. Surgical concerns 9. Psychosocial	1. Nursing physical assessment • Frequent VS • Pain evaluation/Effective pain management • Neurologic assessment – note when awake • Document any signs of neurologic deterioration, LOC, pupillary response, evidence of mental status changes, seizures 3. Frequent monitoring of HR, BP and circulatory status • Maintenance of arterial line, any central venous lines or dialysis catheters if present • Monitor for hypertension related to pain, fluid overload, immunosuppressants • Observe for possible hypotension 4. Nutrition • Consider stomach protection with H2 blocker or proton pump inhibitor for stomach protection when NPO • Early IV or enteral nutrition to support healing • Strict intake and output 5. Serial laboratory studies to include coagulation studies, 6. Positioning, prevention of skin breakdown • Initial and ongoing evaluation of wound site • Observation of potential skin breakdown from devices 7. Expect orders for prophylactic antibiotics and immune suppressants • Evaluate for any signs of allergy, drug–drug interactions or other untoward effects of new medication. • Note and report fever and initial signs of sepsis 8. Surgical postoperative care • Identification and assessment of drains, NG tube, urinary catheter, etc. and wound site

(continued on next page)

Table 3 (continued)	
Critical Care Considerations	Nursing Care Recommendations
	• Post-surgical Assessment for signs of liver dysfunction • First 24 h: nonwakening, bleeding, increasing liver enzymes, lactic acidosis, and shock indicate nonfunction within 24 h • First 48 h: if total bilirubin, coagulation studies, liver function tests not improving 9. Include family members/care providers in discussion of status and planning of care • Encourage family participation in caring for child and continued presence as soon as possible postoperatively • Consult social worker/case manager for counseling and support • Refer to transplant counselor if available • Provide postoperative education and information regarding potential rejection and continued care

* indicates that suggested testing, etc, may be individualized.
  Data from Radovich P. Liver, kidney and pancreas transplantation. In Good VS, Kirkwood PL, eds. *Advanced Critical Care Nursing, 2nd Edition.* 2018, chapter 20:420-435. Elsevier; and Tissieres P, Devictor DJ. Acute liver failure and liver transplantation. In Morrison W, Nelson McMillan KL, Shaffner D. *Rogers Handbook of Pediatric Intensive Care*, 5th edition. 2017: chapter 80:550-554. Wolters Kluwer.

experience constant stress.[34] Parents of children who underwent liver transplantation may have high caregiving burden with low social support systems which did change over time with decreasing caregiving burden and increased social system support.[34]

As a rare illness, with high morbidity and mortality and one with sometimes no explanation for occurrence, PALF poses challenges for both health care providers and families of children whose status can change continually and acutely. Nurses at the bedside are in the best position to provide support for these families and to reinforce the nature of this illness. The need to refer family members to social work or counseling are important additional assessment tasks.

Education for families cannot be overlooked, as this diagnosis may present lifestyle changes affecting diet and activities and continued medical therapy. Children may also be discharged from the hospital awaiting a transplant, with chronic liver failure or post transplant. For those who make a full recovery from PALF, the same concerns do not exist, but the experience of critical illness can have lasting effects. Nurses, along with the multidisciplinary team assist in creating a care plan that aligns the individual needs of the child and appropriate referrals.

Resources for families with children who have chronic liver disease or who have suffered ALF include the American Liver Foundation (Liverfoundation.org), National Organization for Rare Disorders: Children Liver Disease Foundation (https://rarediseases.org/organizations/childrens-liver-disease-foundation/), and the Childhood Liver Disease Research Network (https://childrennetwork.org/)

DISCUSSION

Healthy children who experience acute and critical illness or trauma are extremely resilient, with improvement often occurring at a faster pace as compared to adult patients. PICU stays tend to be shorter and full recovery is likely. This may not be true when children present with or develop fulminant liver failure. It is extremely important to monitor liver function with any type of critical illness, especially with infectious processes and accidental or intentional drug overdose. It is also of utmost importance to refer children with ALF to pediatric centers where transplant services are available as soon as possible. In the United States, there are approximately 250 children's hospitals, but not every state has one nor does every children's hospital have solid organ transplant services. In some areas of the United States, transport services are not easily accessible, so identifying the need for escalation in care should be considered early in the disease process. It takes a team of specialists to provide care who have full and current knowledge of the transplant process, including organ procurement and post-transplant care.

SUMMARY

PALF is a rare, pediatric problem encountered in acute or intensive care. Questions remain regarding etiology, pathology, and treatment. It is important for nurses to consider this potential diagnosis for patients who present to the PICU with a variety of pediatric disorders and to carefully engage in nursing assessment to identify subtle changes following a system-based evaluation approach. Awareness of the trajectory of illness, potential complications, and proposed therapies allows efficient management. Important additions to care include support of the individual child, family members, and care providers early in admission, as this critical diagnosis can present acute as well as life-long effects.

CLINICS CARE POINTS

- Pediatric acute liver failure (PALF) is a rare but significant and potentially life-threatening diagnosis in children.
- Acute liver failure can occur from a variety of causes in a child without previous liver dysfunction, with infection, and acetaminophen toxicity as the primary etiology.
- Critical care nurses are charged with identifying rapid or subtle changes in neurologic status, monitoring hemodynamic patterns, and calculation of fluids through careful intake and output in all critically ill patients, but specifically for those with diagnosed PALF.
- Multisystem organ dysfunction is commonly associated with PALF, requiring frequent assessment, lab monitoring, and life-sustaining treatments including invasive ventilation, continuous renal replacement therapy, high-volume plasmapheresis, and liver transplantation.
- Timely referral for patients with PALF to a pediatric transplant center is one of the most important goals of care.

DISCLOSURE

Both C. Haut and L. Flynn have nothing to disclose. The authors would like to acknowledge Dr Adebowale Adeyemi, gastroenterologist and hepatologist at Nemours Children's Health, who assisted with validating some information in this article.

REFERENCES

1. Berardi G, Tuckfield L, DelVecchio MT, et al. Differential diagnosis of acute liver failure in children: a systematic review. Pediatric Gastroenterology. Hepatol Nutr 2020;23(6):501.
2. Núñez-Ramos R, Montoro S, Bellusci M, et al. Acute liver failure: outcome and value of pediatric end-stage liver disease score in pediatric cases. Pediatr Emerg Care 2018;34(6):409–12.
3. Centers for Disease Control and Prevention (CDC) National Center for Health Statistics. Fast stats: chronic liver disease and cirrhosis. Available at: https://www.cdc.gov/nchs/fastats/liver-disease.htm. Accessed January 24, 2022.
4. Squires JE, Alonso EM, Ibrahim SH, et al. North American Society for pediatric Gastroenterology, Hepatology, and nutrition position paper on the diagnosis and management of pediatric acute liver failure. J Pediatr Gastroenterol Nutr 2022;74(1):138–58.
5. Lutfi R, Abulebda K, Nitu ME, et al. Intensive care management of pediatric acute liver failure. J Pediatr Gastroenterol Nutr 2017;64(5):660–70.
6. Shah NJ, Royer A, John S. Acute liver failure. In: In: StatPearls [Internet]. US National Library of Medicine. Treasure Island (FL: StatPearls Publishing; 2021. Available at: https://www.ncbi.nlm.nih.gov/books/NBK482374/. Accessed January 24, 2021.
7. Squires RH Jr, Shneider BL, Bucuvalas J, et al. Acute liver failure in children: the first 348 patients in the pediatric acute liver study group. J Pediatr 2006;148(5):652–8.
8. Starzl TE, Iwatsuki S, Van Thiel DH, et al. Evolution of liver transplantation. Hepatology 1982;2(5):614–36.
9. Cuenca AG, Kim HB, Vakili K. Pediatric liver transplantation. Semin Pediatr Surg 2017;26(4):217–23. Available at: https://www.ncbi.nlm.nih.gov/pubmed/28964477.
10. Wang KS. Section on surgery; committee on fetus and newborn; childhood liver disease research network. newborn screening for biliary atresia. Pediatrics 2015;136(6):e1663–9.
11. Mysore KR, Shneider BL, Harpavat S. Biliary atresia as a disease starting in utero: implications for treatment, diagnosis and pathogenesis. J Pediatr Gastroenterol Nutr 2019;69(4):396–403.
12. Keles E, Hassan-Kadle MA, Osman MM, et al. Clinical characteristics of acute liver failure associated with hepatitis A infection in children in Mogadishu, Somalia: a hospital-based retrospective study. BMC Infect Dis 2021;21(1):890.
13. Squires J, Alonso E. Acute liver failure in children. In: Suchy FJ, Sokol RJ, Balistreri WF, et al, editors. Liver disease in children. 5th edition. London: Cambridge University Press; 2021. p. 36–57.
14. Fang WY, Abuduxikuer K, Shi P, et al. Pediatric Wilson disease presenting as acute liver failure: prognostic indices. World J Clin Cases 2021;9(14):3273–86.
15. Socha P, Janczyk W, Dhawan A, et al. Wilson's disease in children: a position paper by the Hepatology Committee of the European Society for Paediatric

Gastroenterology, Hepatology and nutrition. J Pediatr Gastroenterol Nutr 2018; 66(2):334–44.

16. Saviano A, Wrensch F, Ghany MG, et al. Liver disease and Coronavirus disease 2019: from pathogenesis to clinical care. Hepatology 2021;74(2):1088–100.

17. Borgi A, Ayari A, Hajji A, et al. Reactivation of human herpes virus 6 and acute liver failure in multisystem inflammatory syndrome. Indian J Pediatr 2021; 88(9):953.

18. Sica R, Pennoni S, Penta L, et al. New onset of hepatic steatosis post-severe multisystem inflammatory syndrome in children (MIS-C): a case report. Int J Environ Res Public Health 2021;18(13):6961.

19. Bulut Y, Sapru A, Roach GD. Hemostatic balance in pediatric acute liver failure: epidemiology of bleeding and thrombosis, physiology and current strategies. Front Pediatr 2020;8:618119.

20. Bolia R, Srivastava A. Recognizing pediatric acute-on-chronic liver failure: the need of the hour. J Pediatr Gastroenterol Nutr 2021;72(1):e29–30.

21. Squires JE, McKeirnan P, Squires RH. Acute liver failure: an update. Clin Liver Dis 2018;22(4):773–804.

22. Flamm SL, Yang YX, Singh S, et al. AGA Institute Clinical Guidelines Committee. American Gastroenterological Association Institute guidelines for the diagnosis and management of acute liver failure. Gastroenterology 2017;152(3):644–7.

23. Bhatt H, Rao GS. Management of acute liver failure: a pediatric perspective. Curr Pediatr Rep 2018;6(3):246–57.

24. Jørgensen MH, Rasmussen A, Christensen VB, et al. Safety of high-volume plasmapheresis in children with acute liver failure. J Pediatr Gastroenterol Nutr 2021; 72(6):815–9.

25. Brar HS, Dadlani A, Ng AM. Successful high-volume plasmapheresis in acute liver failure. Cureus 2021;13(7):e16143.

26. Rawal N, Yazigi N. Pediatric liver transplantation. Pediatr Clin North Am 2017; 64(3):677–84.

27. Children's Oncology Group (COG): in treatment for hepatoblastoma. 2021. Available at: https://childrensoncologygroup.org/in-treatment-with-hepatoblastoma-or-hepatocellular-carcinoma. Accessed: January 26, 2022.

28. Chang CH, Bryce CL, Shneider BL, et al. Accuracy of the Pediatric End-stage Liver Disease score in estimating pretransplant mortality among pediatric liver transplant candidates. JAMA Pediatr 2018;172(11):1070–7.

29. Squires RH, Ng V, Romero R, et al. Evaluation of the pediatric patient for liver transplantation: 2014 practice guideline by the American Association for the Study of Liver Diseases, American Society of Transplantation and the North American Society for Pediatric Gastroenterology, Hepatology and Nutrition. Hepatology 2014;60(1):362–98.

30. Organ Procurement and Transplantation Network (OPTN) US Department of Health and Human Services. Available at: https://optn.transplant.hrsa.gov/. Accessed January 26, 2022.

31. Grek A, Arasi L. Acute liver failure. AACNACConline.org. 2016;27(4):420–9.

32. Bischoff SC, Bernal W, Dasarathy S, et al. ESPEN practical guideline: clinical nutrition in liver disease. Clin Nutr 2020;39(12):3533–62.

33. Abela KM, Wardell D, Rozmus C, et al. Impact of pediatric critical illness and injury on families: an updated systematic review. J Pediatr Nurs 2020;51:21–31.

34. Yayan EH, Düken ME. A comparison of caregiving burden and social support levels of parents of children undergoing liver transplant. J Pediatr Nurs 2019; 47:e45–50.

Hepatitis B and Acute Liver Failure

Nikki Ledoux, BSN, RN

KEYWORDS

- Hepatitis B • Acute liver failure • Hepatitis B reactivation

KEY POINTS

- Reactivation of hepatitis B is associated with the administration of immunosuppressive therapy and the use of direct-acting antivirals to treat hepatitis C treatment in patients with previous exposure to hepatitis B.
- It is imperative to check hepatitis B viral load before, during, and after hepatitis C treatment and immunosuppressive therapy if the patient is at risk for reactivation.
- Early recognition and treatment are imperative for survival of hepatitis B-induced acute liver failure.

At present, viral hepatitis is one of the main causes of acute liver failure (ALF). The most fulminant viral cases are reported after an infection with hepatitis A, B, and B/D. ALF is less often associated with hepatitis C infections. Drug-induced liver injury accounts for greater than 50% of ALF cases.[1] Hepatitis B can cause liver failure due to an acute infection, acute on chronic infection, and reactivation of hepatitis B. Reactivation of hepatitis B can occur in individuals as a complication of chemotherapy or immunosuppressive or biological therapies for the management of rheumatologic conditions, malignancies, inflammatory bowel disease, dermatologic conditions, or solid organ or bone marrow transplantations.[2] The use of direct-acting antiviral medications to treat patients with chronic hepatitis C has resulted in acute hepatitis B and ALF in some patients who were previously exposed to hepatitis B. The ALF resulting from hepatitis B flair in the presence of hepatitis C treatment prompted a black box warning on the new direct-acting antiviral medications and a warning to check hepatitis B serologies before initiating hepatitis C treatment.[3] To better understand hepatitis B in relation to ALF first hepatitis B is discussed.

INTRODUCTION

In 2019 the World Health Organization estimated that 296 million people were infected with the hepatitis B virus (HBV).[4] It is estimated that there are 2.2 million people in the

Southeast Louisiana Veterans Health Care System, Medicine Service Room 3H 124, 2400 Canal Street, New Orleans, LA 70119, USA
E-mail address: Nikki.ledoux@va.gov

Crit Care Nurs Clin N Am 34 (2022) 259–265
https://doi.org/10.1016/j.cnc.2022.04.012
0899-5885/22/Published by Elsevier Inc.

United States with hepatitis B and only a small number of them know they are infected with the HBV.[2] It is estimated that in 2019, 1.5 million people were newly infected with chronic HBV.[4] The HBV is a double-stranded DNA virus that is transmitted percutaneously, sexually, and perinatally. In endemic areas, such as Africa and Asia, it is most often transmitted perinatally.[5] In the Western world HBV is mostly transmitted by reuse of needles and syringes; tattooing; sharing razors; medical, surgical, or dental procedures; and needlesticks among health care workers.[1] HBV can live on a surface for up to 7 days. In endemic areas it is common to see hepatitis B transmitted horizontally/vertically by young children playing and biting or scratching. Hepatitis B has a long incubation period. After initial exposure the average incubation period is 60 days but could be between 28 and 160 days. The presence of the hepatitis B surface antigen (HBsAg) confirms that HBV is present in the blood. The outcome of hepatitis B infection depends on the host immunologic factors and characteristics of the virus; however, age does play a huge role. If the HBV is acquired perinatally at age less than 1 year 80% to 90% develop a chronic infection. If the virus is acquired in children between ages 1 and 5 years, 30% to 50% develop chronic infection. In adults, 30% to 50% are asymptomatic and only 2% to 6% develop chronic infection.[6] The diagnostic criteria for chronic hepatitis B uses hepatitis B serologies to determine the phase of hepatitis B:

- Chronic hepatitis B phase is characterized by the presence of HBsAg for greater than 6 months; in hepatitis B e antigen (HBeAg)-positive cases the HBV viral load typically is greater than 20,000 IU/mL and in HbeAg-negative cases HBV viral load may range from 2000 to 20,000 IU/mL; the alanine aminotransaminase (ALT) and the aspartate aminotransferase (AST) levels can be normal or elevated.
- Immune-tolerant phase of hepatitis B (IT) is characterized by being HBsAg positive for greater than 6 months; HBV viral load can be undetectable or more than several million; in HBeAg-positive individuals, HBV viral levels are usually greater than 20,000 IU/mL and in HBeAg-negative patients, HBV viral levels are usually lower. ALT level can be normal or elevated, as can the AST level
- Immune clearance/active phase of hepatitis B (IA) is characterized by being HBsAg positive for greater than 6 months, HBV viral level greater than 20,000 IU/mL in HBeAg-positive patients, and HBV viral levels greater than 2000 IU/mL in HBeAg-negative patients.
- Inactive carrier phase of hepatitis B (IC) is characterized by being HBsAg positive for greater than 6 months, HBeAg negative, hepatitis B e antibody positive, HBV viral levels less than 2000 IU/mL, and consistently normal ALT and AST levels.[7]

Acute exacerbation can occur in the IA phase (40%–50%). HBsAg can be detected in high levels during acute or chronic infection. The presence of the hepatitis B surface antibody (HBsAb) is interpreted as recovery resulting in immunity from HBV infection. HBsAb is also present in an individual who has successfully been vaccinated. Hepatitis B core antibody (HBcAb) appears in the acute HBV onset phase and remains for life. The presence of the IgM antibody to HBV indicates recent infection with HBV, normally less than 6 months; this indicates acute infection. The acute exacerbation of HBV can lead to ALF.[8]

SYMPTOMS OF HEPATITIS B

The symptoms of hepatitis B are fatigue, fever, muscle aches, joint aches, dark urine, and jaundice.[6] It is also not unusual for adults to be asymptomatic with no detection.[1]

Since the emergence of the antiviral therapies in the 1980s, there has been great progress in the treatment of chronic hepatitis B.[9] HBV can lead to several hepatic complications including acute and chronic hepatitis, cirrhosis, hepatocellular carcinoma, and fulminant liver failure. In acute infections the HBsAg should clear within 3 to 6 months of onset.[6]

In severe acute exacerbation of hepatitis B, the patient often presents with an acute onset of jaundice, and ALT levels that are very high. The patient may complain of nausea, diarrhea, fever, and difficulty concentrating. The patient with severe acute exacerbation of chronic hepatitis B may have positive IgM anti-HBcAb. A comprehensive evaluation of the patient's medical history and review of clinical diagnostic data is imperative to determine the cause of the exacerbation of hepatitis B.[10]

ACUTE LIVER FAILURE

Acute liver injury (ALI) is an assault on the liver characterized by widespread hepatocyte injury. According to the American Association for the Study of Liver Disease (AASLD), ALF is defined as an acute coagulation abnormality, usually an international normalized ratio (INR) greater than 1.5 and any degree of mental alteration (encephalopathy) in a patient without preexisting liver disease.[11] ALF is a clinical syndrome associated with a high rate of mortality if not recognized and treated in a critical care setting preferably in a transplant center.[1]

ALF affects 1600 to 2000 patients per year in the United States. The number of ALF cases related to hepatitis B has declined over the last few decades in the developed countries.[4] Although hepatitis B is responsible for about 7% of cases of ALF in the United States, it remains a problem worldwide.[12] ALF secondary to HBV infection can be related to primoinfection or reactivation of a current or previous infection.[13] In addition, with the use of direct-acting antivirals for the treatment of hepatitis C there have been reports of patients developing a reactivation of hepatitis B. The reactivation of hepatitis B in the presence of hepatitis C treatment has been associated with ALF and has resulted in a liver transplantation in 1 patient and 1 death in another patient.[8] Consideration should be given to treating chronic hepatitis B prophylactically with antiviral therapy before initiating chemotherapy.

CLINICAL MANAGEMENT

The prognosis of ALF due to hepatitis B is poor and in severe cases may require transplantation, therefore treatment with nucleotide analogues should be started immediately.[13] Retrospective clinical trials suggest that antiviral treatment can improve the prognosis of patients with severe forms of acute hepatitis or reactivation including ALF. Thus, nucleotides analogues such as entecavir or tenofovir are treatment options due to their high efficacy.[14] Nucleotide analogues will aid in the suppression of HBV DNA, which will calm down the immune activity and improve the transplant-free survival rate.[5]

All nucleotide analogues carry a black box warning about mitochondrial dysfunction, which normally presents as myopathy, neuropathy, or lactic acidosis. Tenofovir has potential nephrotoxic side effects and bone density loss particularly in patients with HIV. Close monitoring of both kidney function and bone mineral reduction is imperative while patients are on therapy. Entecavir is thought to be associated with lactic acidosis in patients with high model for end-stage liver disease (MELD) scores but has been deemed safe to use in patients with compensated and decompensated cirrhosis. Because hepatitis B often requires lifelong treatment, the long-term safety of the drugs remains one of the most instrumental factors in determining the treatment of choice.[15]

TRANSPLANTATION

Liver transplantation is the single most important intervention to improve the prognosis of hepatitis B-related ALF.[10] Patients who receive a liver transplant have 1- and 5-year survival rates of approximately 84% and 75%, respectively.[14] In patients with immunosuppression-mediated reactivation the possibility of liver transplant is low because of underlying malignant disease.[7] There are several restrictions to liver transplant that should be considered: organ shortage, severe clinical deterioration, severe comorbidities, and substance abuse.[10] The transplant survival rates in ALF due to HBV are lower than liver transplants survival rates for other indications. Based on the analysis of the United Network for Organ Sharing, factors that impact survival rates are recipient age greater than 50 years, the requirement for life support, a body mass index greater than or equal to 30 kg/m^2, and a serum creatinine level greater than 2.0 mg/dL. Additional factors that are associated with a poor prognosis are the use of a liver that is too small for the recipient, donor age greater than 60 years, incompatible ABO group matching, and donor livers with steatosis.[14]

SUPPORTIVE CARE

Supportive treatment of ALF is essential and requires close monitoring of hemodynamic state and aggressive treatment of complications by a multidisciplinary team; this is typically done in the intensive care setting preferably in a transplant center. A comprehensive physical assessment is essential and should include assessment of neurologic and mental status. For patients with severe encephalopathy airway management may be needed including intubation. Infections are treated with antibiotics, whereas coagulability may be treated with transfusions.[5]

Most patients with ALF due to HBV present with inadequate intake and malnutrition. Liver failure results in portal hypertensive gastropathy, portal hypertensive enteropathy, increased abdominal pressure, and intestinal flora disorders leading to malnutrition. Nutritional support started at admission has demonstrated better patient outcomes.[16]

Hemodynamic stability should be assessed, and intravenous fluids administered for electrolyte imbalance. Patients with ALF usually present with hyperdynamic circulation. Correcting fluid imbalance is essential to improve tissue perfusion. Vasopressors and inotropic drugs may be used to maintain arterial pressure and cardiac output. Hemodynamic monitoring is essential to choose the proper intervention without adverse effects.[17–19]

Ventilator support may be needed for patients with impaired consciousness or those who develop acute respiratory distress syndrome (ARDS). In patients with ALF about 21% develop ARDS, which is usually associated with sepsis.[14] Although the development of ARDS suggests more days on mechanical ventilation, there is no difference in intensive care unit days or in mortality.[14]

Acute kidney injury (AKI) is seen in up to 70% of patients with 30% requiring renal replacement therapy (RRT).[14] AKI is associated with decreased survival. If needed, RRT should be continuous rather than intermittent to improve the hemodynamic state and decrease the risk of cerebral ischemia.[14]

As a result of immune system dysfunction patients with ALF are at increased risk for infections and sepsis leading to an increased risk of mortality. Bacterial infections have been reported in 80% of cases. Active surveillance for infections is necessary because the mortality attributed to sepsis is between 10% and 52%. The most common infections are pneumonia, urinary tract infections, and bloodstream infections. Multiresistant infections play a significant role in these patients. Fungal infections affect up to one-third of the cases.[14]

Routine blood culture and the administration of broad-spectrum antibiotics are recommended if the patient's clinical picture worsens. However, the benefits of antibiotic prophylaxis are controversial, and the exact antimicrobial should be based on local microbiological data.[14]

The synthesis of coagulation factors, anticoagulation factors, and fibrinolytic system are diminished in ALF. Although an increased INR is an important prognostic factor, it is not an indication of a risk for hemorrhage. Platelet counts are reduced, and there is abnormal platelet function.[14]

Bleeding in patients with acute liver disease can occur spontaneously. The most common site of bleeding in patients with acute liver disease is the gastric mucosa. Therefore, proton pump inhibitors are recommended. It is essential to evaluate the homeostatic balance and make necessary corrections before performing procedures to manage the bleeding. Prophylactic blood component transfusions based on conventional coagulation assays are not recommended.[14]

It is critical to recognize intracranial hypertension (ICH) early because it accounts for 20% to 35% of mortality in ALF. Frequent neurologic assessments are necessary to avoid permanent neurologic damage. ICH is a pressure greater than 20 to 25 mm Hg for more than 15 minutes. ICH is attributed to the poor metabolization of ammonia by the hepatocytes leading to an accumulation of glutamine in astrocytes, which yields an osmotic effect and leads to cellular edema, encephalopathy, and eventually ICH. There is vasodilatation of the cerebral arterioles leading to intracranial blood volume. The diagnosis of ICH is based on continuous neurologic assessments, periodic neuroimaging, and intracranial pressure monitoring.[13] Although hepatic encephalopathy is associated with ICH, additional risk factors for ICH are female gender, younger age, severe liver failure with a MELD score greater than 32, ammonia concentrations higher than 150 to 200 μmol/L, and renal failure.[14]

SUMMARY

Although hepatitis B-related ALF is an infrequent condition, it is essential for clinicians to recognize the syndrome and intervene promptly. The incidence of hepatitis B ALF is 1 to 8 cases per million inhabitants, and it has a poor prognosis and high mortality. The management of the patient is best done by a multidisciplinary team of health care providers preferably in a transplant center. The intensive care nursing staff is the most qualified to monitor and provide the necessary care. Encouraging vaccination for HBV is one strategy to decrease the number of hepatitis B-related ALF cases.

The hepatitis B vaccination is effective and generates protective levels of antibodies in 95% of children and 90% of adults. Revaccination is effective in 80% of individuals who do not respond to the first series. In neonates of hepatitis B-positive mothers, it is important to vaccinate within 24 hours of birth. If the vaccine is given after 7 days, there is no evidence of postexposure protection.[6]

Any patient with liver disease should receive the hepatitis B and A vaccines. Other individuals who should receive hepatitis B vaccines are those with HIV, those who are immunocompromised, health care workers, sexual partners of hepatitis B-positive individuals, and individuals on hemodialysis.[10] Once vaccinated, patients on hemodialysis should have their hepatitis B antibodies checked annually because their immunity can decrease. If the hepatitis B antibody titers are low, less than 10 IU/mL, a booster is recommended.[7]

CASE STUDY

A 75-year-old man with chronic hepatitis B was not on an antiviral because he did not meet AASLD criteria to treat. His blood work was HBsAg positive, HBcAb positive, HBsAb negative, and viral load detectable but not quantifiable. The result of his liver function test was within normal range.

He was diagnosed with mantle cell non-Hodgkins lymphoma stage IV with central nervous system involvement. He was started on chemotherapy. At the same time he was started on chemotherapy he was started on entecavir 300 mg daily. He did well for 2 years. The cancer responded to chemotherapy, and the chemotherapy was discontinued. Entecavir was also discontinued.

Within 2 months, the patient called the clinic complaining of fatigue, loss of appetite, general malaise, and nausea. He was seen in clinic. At the time of his clinic visit, he appeared jaundiced upon examination and he was noted to have newly developed ascites. Blood work was done. The results were total bilirubin 7.8 mg/dl, AST 2519 IU/L, ALT 1721 IU/L, albumin 2.8 g/dl, alkaline phosphatase 157 IU/L, and INR 1.9. The patient had stopped his entecavir and was experiencing a reactivation of his hepatitis B. The patient was experiencing an acute on chronic hepatitis B flair.

He was transported from clinic to a transplant center for care. There his entecavir was restarted. He responded well to treatment without a transplant. The antiviral was continued indefinitely.

CLINICS CARE POINTS

- Initiate hepatitis B vaccine series at birth.
- Check hepatitis B serologies before starting immunosuppressant medication. Initiate treatment of HBV if necessary.
- Check hepatitis B serologies before initiating hepatitis C therapy, vaccinate if necessary. Treat for HBV if necessary.
- Continue hepatitis B antivirals for 6 months after discontinuing immunosuppressants and 12 months after discontinuing B cell-depleting agents.
- Medical history can aid in determining reactivation of acute hepatitis B.

DISCLOSURE

The author has nothing to disclose.

REFERENCES

1. Manka P, Verheyen J, Guido G, et al. Liver failure due to acute viral hepatitis (A-E). Visc Med 2016;32:80–5.
2. Loomba R, Liang T. Hepatitis B reactivation associated associated with immune suppressive and biological Modifier therapies: current concepts management Strategies, and Future direction. Gastroenterology 2017;152:1297–309.
3. Pockros P. Black box warning for possible HBV reactivation during DAA therapy for chronic HCV infection. Gastroenterol Hepatol 2017;13(9):536–40.

4. World Health Organization. Global progress report on HIV, viral hepatitis and sexually transmitted infections. 2021. Available at. https://www.who.int/publications/:/item/9789240027077.
5. Wong V, Chan H. Severe acute exacerbation of chronic hepatitis B: a unique presentation of a common disease. J Gastroenterol Hepatol 2009;24:1179–86.
6. Heathcote J, Elewaut A, Fedail S, et al. World Gastroenterology Organization Practice Guidelines: management of acute viral hepatitis. World Gastroenterol Organ 2007;1–13.
7. Terrault N, Lok A, McMahon B, et al. Update on Prevention diagnosis and treatment of chronic hepatitis B: AASLD 2018 hepatitis B Guidance. Hepatology 2018;67(4).
8. Li Q, Wang J, Lu M, et al. Acute-on-Chronic liver failure from chronic- hepatitis-B, who is the behind the Scenes. Front Microbiol 2020;11:583423.
9. Feng Z, Li Y. Nursing interventions in hepatitis B patient care[thesis]. Jyvaskyla, Finland: JAMK University of Applied Sciences; 2020.
10. Sedano R, Castro L, Venegas M, et al. Liver transplantation in acute liver failure due to Hepatitis B. Two clinical cases. Ann Hepatol 2021;100107.
11. Kwong S, Meyerson C, Zheng W, et al. Acute hepatitis and acute liver failure: Pathologic diagnosis and differential diagnosis. Semin Diagn Pathol 2019;36:404–14.
12. Sedhom D, D'Souza M, John E, et al. Viral hepatitis and acute liver failure: Still a problem. Clin Liver Dis 2018;22:289–300.
13. Oketani M, Uto H, Ido A, et al. Management of hepatitis B virus-related acute liver failure. Clin J Gastroenterol 2014;7:19–26.
14. Rovengo M, Magdalena V, Ruiz A, et al. Current concepts in acute liver failure. Ann Hepatol 2019;18:543–52.
15. Kayaaslan B, Guner R. Adverse effects of oral antiviral therapy in chronic Hepatis B. World J Hepatol 2017;9:227–41.
16. Chang Y, Liu Q, Zhang Q, et al. Role of nutritional status and nutritional support in outcome of hepatitis B virus-associated acute-on-chronic liver failure. World J Gastroenterol 2020;26:4288–301.
17. Shah NJ, Royer A, John S. Acute liver failure. [Updated 2021 Jul19]. In: Stat-Pearls [Internet]. Treasure Island (FL): StatPearls Publishing; 2022. Available at: https://www.ncbi.nlm.nih.gov/books/NBK482374/.
18. Kappus M, Sterling R. Extrahepatic Manifestations of acute hepatitis B virus infection. Gastroenterol Hepatol 2013;9:123–6.
19. Wang C, Zhao P, Liu W, et al. Acute liver failure caused by severe acute hepatitis B: a case series from a multi-center investigation. Ann Clin Microbiol Antimicrobials 2014;13:23.

Drug-Induced Liver Injury

Cathy McAtee, DNP, CCRN, ACNP-BC, CNE

KEYWORDS

- Hepatotoxicity • Drug-induced liver injury • DILI
- Idiosyncratic drug-induced liver injury • Liver injury patterns

KEY POINTS

- Drug-induced liver injury (DILI) can be further characterized by latency, drug exposure, bilirubin, ALT, and alkaline phosphatase levels.
- DILI with some drugs has a therapeutic treatment option but most cases involve the cessation of the drug and supportive care.
- Idiosyncratic drug reactions are unpredictable and complicate the drug trials, drug approval process, and the cost of drug development.

Clinicians often encounter drug-induced liver injury (DILI) when caring for patients in an acute care setting. Damage to the liver's hepatocytes can be caused by the drug, the drug's metabolites or a hypersensitivity response involving the innate and adaptive immune system.[1] Prompt recognition and removal of offending agent(s) in patients with clinical signs of DILI can prevent a pathologic progression of injury that could result in acute liver failure (ALF) or chronic impairment of liver function.[2] Clinicians strive to uphold the goal that all care delivered will "do no harm." In reality, iatrogenic hepatic injury constitutes at least one-third of the renowned Hepatotoxicity text authored by Hyman Zimmerman, who highlighted the numerous clinical manifestations of DILI across drug classes. DILI is a complex interaction between genetic, environmental, pharmacologic, and possible herbal factors that is difficult to predict in most cases. DILI affects 20 persons per 100,000 of the population each year[3] and only 30% of those cases are accompanied by jaundice[4,5] and many silent subclinical presentations are discovered in routine laboratory analysis.[6] Because DILI mimics acute and chronic forms of hepatic disease,[7] knowledge of the general principles, phenotypes, mechanisms, and usual drug suspects can help differentiate the etiology of hepatocellular toxicity of DILI from other causes of liver disease. DILI is the most common reason for nonapproval of new drugs, withdrawal from the market, black box warnings, and other regulatory actions[6] that contribute to the exorbitant cost of pharmaceutical research and new drug development.

Adult Gerontology, Acute Care Nurse Practitioner Program, Louisiana Health Science Center – New Orleans, 1900 Gravier Street, Suite 156, New Orleans, LA 70112, USA
E-mail address: cmcat2@lsuhsc.edu

Crit Care Nurs Clin N Am 34 (2022) 267–275
https://doi.org/10.1016/j.cnc.2022.04.007
0899-5885/22/Published by Elsevier Inc.

ccnursing.theclinics.com

HISTORY

Drug hepatotoxicity received early recognition and research by Dr Hyman Zimmerman in 1948 while he was working with the Veterans Administration and found this venue to be conducive to his interest in DILI and hepatology.[8] Dr Zimmerman's interest in hepatology began during World War II when he cared for GIs suffering from an unknown hepatic malady, now known as hepatitis A. His early work delineated a system for defining hepatic injury that is still used today by modern medicine and that helped to create the subspecialty of hepatology.[9] The classification system Dr Zimmerman developed to describe DILI was later refined by the Council for International Medical Sciences and the Food and Drug Administration (FDA.[2]; Dr Zimmerman frequently stated, "Drug-induced hepatocellular jaundice is a serious lesion, with mortality from 10% to 50%,"[10] p. 19). The FDA modified this statement and titled it Hy's law (also known as Hy's rule) to describe the relationship between jaundice without obstruction and death in 10% to 50% of DILI cases. Dr Zimmerman's observations of DILI resulted in removing harmful medications from clinical practice and retaining medications for which the therapeutic benefit outweighs the risk of hepatotoxicity.[11]

DEFINITIONS

ALF is a sudden onset of severe liver injury accompanied by coagulopathy as evidenced by international normalized ratio ≥ 1.5 and signs and symptoms of hepatic encephalopathy with no previous history of cirrhosis or other liver disease.[12]

DILI is damage to hepatocytes and other liver cells sustained in the metabolism of xenobiotics.[13]

Xenobiotics are substances that are not produced or expected within an organism and provide an extrinsic exposure to the organism.[14–16] Xenobiotics include both prescription and over-the-counter medications, vitamins, supplements, herbs, and other substances ingested both intentionally and unintentionally.

Cytochrome P450 (CYP) is a large group of enzymes found in nearly all forms of life to assist with the metabolism of endogenous and exogenous compounds. The CYP superfamily includes the most well-known drug-metabolizing enzymes present in the liver with CPY 1, CPY 2 & CPY 3 responsible for 80% of clinical drug metabolism.[17]

Biotransformation is a process of detoxification of xenobiotics through a series of phases in which xenobiotics are converted to substances that are more easily eliminated by the body[18]; it generally has a series of detoxification mechanisms from phase 0 to phase 3.[19]

BACKGROUND

One of the liver's major functions is to detoxify xenobiotics, but during this process, biotransformation of these substances can induce unintended liver injury along multiple pathways. Most drugs that cause DILI have a unique characteristic of latent, pathologic, and clinical profiles, but some hepatoxic drugs present with multiple or mixed profiles.[7] The liver is particularly susceptible to harm during the biotransformation of substances that have been ingested in the gastrointestinal (GI) tract.[13] The most preferred route of drug delivery is oral as dosing is easy and painless, and this type of drug is cost-effective to manufacture. Conditions in the GI tract such as pH, long gastric emptying time, food effects, and first-pass metabolism reduce the bioavailability of most orally consumed drugs. Most drugs are largely metabolized in the first pass mechanism long before the drug reaches its target site as blood is delivered a short distance between the intestinal lumen and the liver via the portal veins. Dosing of oral drugs is much higher to allow for this significant reduction in bioavailability as a result of the first-pass metabolism.[20] The list of drugs that could cause DILI is extensive and includes such classes as antimicrobials, antifungals, antitumor, immunosuppressants, antivirals, and many miscellaneous drugs.[1] The impact of hepatoxicity can range from rarely (eg, <1% per 50,000 cases for statin drugs) to often (eg, 0.1%–1% of individuals treated with isoniazid). Of the 1089 patients that were deemed to be highly likely, or probable to suffer from DILI in the DILIN trial, 9.8% were referred for liver transplant or died. Most of the patients with ALF in the DILIN prospective trial were referred for liver transplantation and 68% of patients with ALF received a transplant. Patients who did not survive were identified as being older, having underlying chronic liver disease, and have a hepatocellular pattern type liver injury.[21] This percentage is consistent with multiple large DILI registries as part of postmarketing surveillance and reporting to regulatory agencies.[13] DILI may also have been a major contributor to other deaths in the trial but was not listed as the primary cause of death.[21]

As part of the FDA's oversight, increased attention is paid to prescription causes of DILI, resulting in an increase in the identification of DILI secondary to over-the-counter herbal and dietary supplements (HDS) in recent years.[13] Many over-the-counter HDS products are poorly regulated and marketed with no scientific evidence of benefit despite their claims to improve health, vitality, and mood. Asian countries have a higher proportion of HDS products and report that greater than 70% of DILI cases are due to them.[2] Patients assume that these nonregulated or natural compounds are harmless and may fail to report their use to the health care provider. There is mounting evidence of harm in the form of hepatocellular pattern DILI, yet their appeal to consumers continues to grow with the highest rates in the United States at greater than 64% of American adults.[22]

There has been an increase in research interest related to the biomarkers for the identification of DILI, genetic predisposition, and prognosis,[23] but more research is needed to identify areas for medical intervention to reduce mortality and the need for subsequent liver transplant. Advances in technology in areas such as pharmacogenomics and toxicogenomics may provide benefits during drug development to reduce the incidence of DILI in the future.[7]

DIRECT INJURY

Direct injury, aka "intrinsic" injury is the most common type of DILI[4]; it is predictable, dose dependent and occurs promptly after ingestion.[13] Although hepatocyte stress can be seen in many patients with high dose exposures, only a small number of them with low immune tolerance of the liver will develop DILI.[1] The mechanism of cell death in direct injury may be related to organelle stress of the endoplasmic reticulum and mitochondria, resulting in multiple distinct pathways of necrosis or apoptosis causing cell death. Apoptosis can take one of the 2 pathways, either the initiation of death receptors in extrinsic apoptosis or intrinsic apoptosis via the permeabilization of the mitochondrial outer membrane; both pathways result in the activation of caspase 3&7.[6]

The most common type of direct injury pattern is associated with acetaminophen overdose, which unfortunately results in ALF[13] and greater than 100,000 calls annually to poison control centers.[6] Approximately 50% of ALF in the United States is attributed to intentional and unintentional acetaminophen overdose.[23] Unintentional overdose can occur at doses that are only marginally above the 4-g per day dose limit, and other confounding factors such as alcohol use, fasting, coexisting disease and other drug ingestion can lower the threshold of toxicity.[13] **Tables 1** and **2** gives a brief overview of medications associated with direct DILI.

Table 1
TNFα inhibitors vs checkpoint inhibitors

Drug Class	Latency	Typical Agents	ALT	ALP	Bili	Comments
TNFα inhibitors	Days to Months	Infliximab Etanercept Adalimumab	Variable	Variable	Variable	Infliximab is more common Hepatocellular and cholestatic injury patterns
Check point inhibitors		Ipilimumab Nivolumab Pembrolizumab	Variable	Variable	Variable	Hepatocellular injury Immune mediated liver injury

Adapted from Shah et al. 2020.

INDIRECT INJURY

With the increasing popularity of prescribing biologics for chronic inflammatory diseases, the rising incidence of DILI has been observed as well. Both TNFα inhibitors and checkpoint inhibitors have been associated with an immune-mediated liver injury that is quite different from other DILI mechanisms. The precise pathway of injury is unknown, but DILI is believed to be the sequelae of immune-mediated hepatitis. Most of the patients affected will recover after removal of the offending agent and the administration of corticosteroids, but some have developed ALF requiring liver transplantation.[24]

IDIOSYNCRATIC DRUG-INDUCED LIVER INJURY

Idiosyncratic drug-induced injury (IDILI) is much more complex, and several speculative theories exist about the adaptive immune system role in injury common to each of the theories.[6] In the United States, IDILI accounts for 11% of ALF cases. IDILI is based on rare cases of individual hypersensitivities to drugs related to reactive metabolites that have been bioactivated by liver enzymes. These include cytochrome P450.[25] IDILI can be further categorized as IDILI with or without immune-allergic features of rash and eosinophilia; most cases are without these immune-allergic features.[6] The cascade

Table 2
Comparison of IDILI phenotypes

IDILI Phenotype	Latency	Typical Agents	ALT	ALK p	Bilirubin	Comments
Acute hepatitis	Days to months	Isoniazid, diclofenac	↑↑↑	↑		High death rate
Cholestatic hepatitis	Weeks to months	Amoxicillin-clavulanate, cefazolin	↑↑↑	↑		Pruritus
Mixed hepatitis	Days to months	Trimethoprim-sulfamethoxazole	↑↑			Self-limiting, usually benign
Chronic hepatitis	Months to years	Diclofenac, nitrofurantoin, minocycline	↑↑		↑	Insidious onset

of injury occurs with typical drug dosing and is not related to overdose.[23] A minimal dose, variable for each individual, is necessary to induce the injury pattern.[13] This type of injury is not reproducible in animal studies and is neither predictable nor dose dependent.[4] Animals used in drug development are also prone to IDILI.[25] The most common type of idiosyncratic DILI is associated with the use of antimicrobials,[2] but it is unclear as to whether the cause is secondary to drug metabolites or disruption of the immune tolerance as a result of alterations in gut flora.[26] In fact, the top 5 drugs in the American DILI Network prospective study (DILIN) were in the antimicrobial drug class, listed as amoxicillin-clavulanate, isoniazid, nitrofurantoin, trimethoprim-sulfamethoxazole and minocycline, and comprised 45.4% of DILI cases. In the United States, HDS have been implicated in approximately 16% of reported cases.[2]

The classification of IDILI is based on the ratio of ALT to alkaline phosphatase (ALP) in relation to the upper limit of normal (ULN) values (**Table 3**).[25]

RISK FACTORS FOR DRUG-INDUCED LIVER INJURY

Research has identified multiple risk factors to identify persons prone to developing DILI. Most interesting is the fact that preexisting liver disease does not increase the risk of DILI.[11] Women in the United States are more inclined to be affected compared with men (59% vs 41%), and women are more susceptible to hepatocellular patterns of injury while men are more susceptible to cholestatic DILI.[2] Advanced age in a European study was found to have 3 times higher rate of DILI but that may be related to the number of prescriptions consumed[2] and greater age predisposes one to cholestatic DILI of a longer course.[6]

Human leukocyte antigen haplotypes associated with chromosome 6[1] may interact with reactive metabolites, placing susceptible persons at risk for DILI[27] through T cell-

Table 3 Injury patterns		
Injury Patterns	**Features**	**Examples**
Hepatocellular injury	ALT ≥ 3times ULN &ALT/ALP ratio >5 times ULN	Antitumor necrosis factor agents Green tea extract Inhaled anesthetics Interferon alpha Interferon beta Isoniazid Lamotrigine Macrolides Minocycline Nitrofurantoin NSAIDS Proton pump inhibitors Valproate
Cholestatic injury	ALP ≥ 2 times ULN & ALT/ALP ratio ≤ 2 times ULN	Amoxicillin-clavulanate Anabolic steroids
Hepatocellular-cholestatic mixed injury	ALT≥3 times ULN, ALP≥2 times the ULN & ALT/ALP ratio<5 but >2 times the ULN	Allopurinol Amiodarone Azathioprine Carbamazepine Fluoroquinolones Phenytoin

mediated and adaptive immune responses.[25] Polymorphisms of other immune-related genes such as variants of protein tyrosine phosphate nonreceptor type 22 (PTPN22) and allele variations of interleukin 10 may also increase the risk.

DRUG DEVELOPMENT

Idiosyncratic DILI may be discovered late in drug development or even after marketing[25] with 46% of drugs prescribed having at least one case report of being the cause of liver injury.[4] DILI is the leading cause of the withdrawal of drugs during drug trial development[1] and of issuing warnings for use.[2] Hepatotoxicity was the cause of 32% of drug withdrawals in the years 1975 to 2007; since the FDA published "Drug Induced Liver Injury: Premarketing Clinical Evaluation," no withdrawals have been attributed to DILI.[13]

DISCUSSION

LiverTox is a National Institute of Health (NIH) website that has cataloged more than 1200 substances that are toxic to the liver, including medications, herbal remedies, supplements, and toxins.[4] This website is updated regularly and is a wealth of unbiased information for the clinician's immediate use.

Recent advances in diagnostic laboratory studies useful for the identification of hepatitis such as PCR technology, genetic mutations in iron overload, and E phosphatidylethanol and ANA are indirectly useful in the diagnosis of DILI when other etiologies are ruled out, making DILI a diagnosis of exclusion[27] Currently there are no reliable in vitro laboratory assays that can predict a drug's likelihood of producing an idiosyncratic reaction.[25] There are multiple hepatic cell models currently being used to evaluate the various mechanisms of DILI in vitro that may be useful in early-stage drug development. These models include the human hepatocyte culture, human pluripotent stem cells, and cell lines derived from hepatomas (hepatocellular carcinomas), but these research methods are deemed unreliable in consistently predicting DILI.[28]

SPECIAL POPULATIONS

The complex drug regimens associated with antituberculosis therapy place some patients at a higher risk of DILI than the general population. In a recent study. DILI is a frequent cause of treatment interruption and morbidity in the tuberculosis patient population. Older patients and those of Asian descent receiving standard antituberculosis drug therapy are at a higher risk of liver enzyme elevations. Isoniazid can be excluded in some cases in a liver-sparing strategy by the substitution of moxifloxacin when necessary.[29] Patients at the highest risk for developing DILI are those living with HIV and coinfected with tuberculosis, 1/3 of these patients develop DILI.[30]

Hepatotoxicity is a common occurrence during chemotherapy and frequently causes delays, dose reductions, and discontinuation of therapy. Antioxidant therapy has been shown to be effective in reducing oxidative stress and liver injury in animal models and may provide a liver protective strategy in some chemotherapy regimens.[31]

CLINICAL MANAGEMENT

If a patient is suspected of having DILI with acutely elevated biomarkers and normal imaging, compare any recent ingestions of xenobiotics with the LiverTox registry at https//www.ncbi.nlm.nih.gov/books/NBK547852/. A careful history of ingestion is needed to identify prescription drugs, illicit drugs, or HDS that could be considered a suspected culprit. Discontinue or "dechallenge" suspected xenobiotics and exclude other causes such as hepatitis, cytomegalovirus, Epstein–Barr virus. Check antinuclear antibodies, antismooth muscle antibody, and IgG. Consider hospitalization and serial monitoring of liver functions and INR and follow this patient until the final disposition. N-Acetylcysteine can be used early in the case of IDILI with ALF. Steroids may benefit patients who have been affected by drugs that have an autoimmune-like clinical presentation (ALT, AST > ALP) positive ANA, and elevated IgG. If the patient presents with moderate to severe abdominal pain, choledocholithiasis needs to be ruled out by MRCP. Viral hepatitis should be ruled out in all patients with acute hepatocellular injury. There is a useful RUCAM worksheet on the LiverTox website that can help determine causality based on onset, dechallenge results, and exclude other etiologies for the hepatic injury pattern.[27] Prompt recognition of DILI, a thorough assessment, and effective monitoring can reduce the incidence of permanent liver damage secondary to DILI. In most cases, discontinuing the offending drug will return the liver to its normal functional state.[7]

SUMMARY

DILI can be direct or idiosyncratic in nature and further characterization can be performed by laboratory analysis of ALT, ALP, and bilirubin. Other causes for liver dysfunction should be explored and ruled out before DILI is considered. A careful history, physical and diagnostic work up is needed to assess latency and injury patterns. Treatment is based on the offending agent and may include referral for liver transplantation, adequate resources are available through LiverTox and the RUCAM causality worksheet to assist the clinicians in caring for this patient population. HDS are products that make up a multibillion-dollar market that is marketing drugs with no scientific proof of benefit and a burgeoning level of evidence of harm. Patients are less likely to disclose the use of HDS products, so a careful and complete history is needed in this DILI patient population to identify DILI secondary to over-the-counter products. Most patients affected with DILI will recover, but approximately 10% will not survive or will be referred for liver transplant. Patients who are older, have underlying chronic liver disease, or have a hepatocellular pattern are the least likely to survive DILI.

CLINICS CARE POINTS

- Cessation of suspected drug
- Administer m-acetylcysteine early in acetaminophen overdose
- Administer corticosteroids for indirect DILI from TNFα or checkpoint inhibitors
- Obtain liver function studies for any patient with itching, rash, nausea, or jaundice
- Obtain liver and biliary imaging, MRCP if indicated
- Rule out hepatitis A, B, C, E CMV, EBV, and HSV
- Check ANA, SMA, IgG
- Rule out alcohol-induced liver disease and recent hypotension
- Serial laboratory analysis
- Consider hospitalization, liver biopsy, and advanced imaging

DISCLOSURE

The author has no financial disclosures or other conflicts of interest.

REFERENCES

1. Ye H, Nelson LJ, Moral M, et al. Dissecting the molecular pathophysiology of drug-induced liver injury. World J Gastroenterol 2018;24(13):1373–85. https://doi.org/10.3748/wjg.v24.i13.1373.
2. Katarey D, Verma S. Drug-induced liver injury. Clin Med 2016;16(Suppl 6): s104–9. https://doi.org/10.7861/clinmedicine.16-6-s104.
3. Leise MD, Poterucha JJ, Talwalkar JA. Drug-induced liver injury. Mayo Clinic Proc 2014;89(1):95–106. https://doi.org/10.1016/j.mayocp.2013.09.016.
4. Hoofnagle JH, Björnsson ES. Drug-induced liver injury — types and phenotypes. N Engl J Med 2019;381(3):264–73. https://doi.org/10.1056/nejmra1816149.
5. Hyman j. zimmerman, md. JAMA 2000;283(6):812. https://doi.org/10.1001/jama.283.6.812.
6. Iorga A, Dara L, Kaplowitz N. Drug-induced liver injury: cascade of events leading to cell death, apoptosis or necrosis. Int J Mol Sci 2017;18(5):1018. https://doi.org/10.3390/ijms18051018.
7. Kaplowitz N. Drug-induced liver injury. Clin Infect Dis 2004;38(Supplement_2): S44–8. https://doi.org/10.1086/381446.
8. Lewis JH, Seeff LB. The origins of the modern-day study of drug hepatotoxicity: focus on hyman j. zimmerman. Clin Liver Dis 2020;15(S1). https://doi.org/10.1002/cld.856.
9. Seef LB. Hyman J. Zimmerman M.D. JAMA 2000;283(6):812.
10. Pauls LL, Senior JR. Drug Induced Liver Injury. FDA Clinical Investigator Training Course 2012.
11. Zimmerman H. Hepatotoxicity. 2nd edition. Amsterdam, Netherlands: Lippencott Williams & Wilkins; 1999.
12. Mendizabal M. Liver transplantation in acute liver failure: a challenging scenario. World J Gastroenterol 2016;22(4):1523. https://doi.org/10.3748/wjg.v22.i4.1523.
13. Andrade RJ, Chalasani N, Björnsson ES, et al. Drug-induced liver injury. Nat Rev Dis Primers 2019;5(1). https://doi.org/10.1038/s41572-019-0105-0.
14. Croom E. Metabolism of xenobiotics of human environments. In: Progress in molecular biology and translational science. Elsevier; 2012. p. 31–88. https://doi.org/10.1016/b978-0-12-415813-9.00003-9.
15. Drug-induced liver injury — types and phenotypes. N Engl J Med 2019;381(14): 1395–6. https://doi.org/10.1056/nejmc1911063.
16. Fontana RJ, Watkins PB, Bonkovsky HL, et al. Drug-induced liver injury network (dilin) prospective study. Drug Saf 2009;32(1):55–68. https://doi.org/10.2165/00002018-200932010-00005.
17. Song Y, Li C, Liu G, et al. Drug-metabolizing cytochrome p450 enzymes have multifarious influences on treatment outcomes. Clin Pharmacokinet 2021;60(5): 585–601. https://doi.org/10.1007/s40262-021-01001-5.
18. Almazroo O, Miah M, Venkataramanan R. Drug metabolism in the liver. Clin Liver Dis 2017;21(1):1–20. https://doi.org/10.1016/j.cld.2016.08.001.
19. Marin JG, Serrano MA, Monte MJ, et al. Role of genetic variations in the hepatic handling of drugs. Int J Mol Sci 2020;21(8):2884. https://doi.org/10.3390/ijms21082884.
20. Patel R, Barker J, ElShaer A. Pharmaceutical excipients and drug metabolism: a mini-review. Int J Mol Sci 2020;21(21):8224. https://doi.org/10.3390/ijms21218224.

21. Hayashi PH, Rockey DC, Fontana RJ, et al. Death and liver transplantation within 2 years of onset of drug-induced liver injury. Hepatology 2017;66(4):1275–85. https://doi.org/10.1002/hep.29283.
22. Grewal P, Ahmad J. Severe liver injury due to herbal and dietary supplements and the role of liver transplantation. World J Gastroenterol 2019;25(46):6704–12. https://doi.org/10.3748/wjg.v25.i46.6704.
23. McGill MR, Jaeschke H. Biomarkers of drug-induced liver injury. In Advances in pharmacology. Elsevier; 2019. p. 221–39. https://doi.org/10.1016/bs.apha.2019.02.001.
24. Shah P, Sundaram V, Björnsson E. Biologic and checkpoint inhibitor-induced liver injury: a systematic literature review. Hepatol Commun 2020;4(2):172–84. https://doi.org/10.1002/hep4.1465.
25. Jee A, Sernoskie S, Uetrecht J. Idiosyncratic drug-induced liver injury: mechanistic and clinical challenges. Int J Mol Sci 2021;22(6):2954. https://doi.org/10.3390/ijms22062954.
26. Rathi, Kumar. 2019.
27. Björnsson ES. Clinical management of patients with drug-induced liver injury (dili). United Eur Gastroenterol J 2021;9(7):781–6. https://doi.org/10.1002/ueg2.12113.
28. Kuna L, Bozic I, Kizivat T, et al. Models of drug induced liver injury (dili) – current issues and future perspectives. Curr Drug Metab 2018;19(10):830–8. https://doi.org/10.2174/1389200219666180523095355.
29. Tweed C, Wills G, Crook AM, et al. Liver toxicity associated with tuberculosis chemotherapy in the remoxtb study. BMC Med 2018;16(1). https://doi.org/10.1186/s12916-018-1033-7.
30. Naidoo K, Hassan-Moosa R, Mlotshwa P, et al. High rates of drug-induced liver injury in people living with hiv coinfected with tuberculosis (tb) irrespective of antiretroviral therapy timing during antituberculosis treatment: results from the starting antiretroviral therapy at three points in tb trial. Clin Infect Dis 2019;70(12):2675–82. https://doi.org/10.1093/cid/ciz732.
31. Vincenzi B, Russo A, Terenzio A, et al. The use of same in chemotherapy-induced liver injury. Crit Rev Oncol Hematol 2018;130:70–7. https://doi.org/10.1016/j.critrevonc.2018.06.019.

HELLP Syndrome

Marie Adorno, PhD, APRN, CNS, RNC-MNN, CNE[a],*,
Cathy Maher-Griffiths, DNS, RN, NEA-BC, RNC-OB[b],
Heather Rose Grush Abadie, DNP, RNC-OB[c]

KEYWORDS

- HELLP syndrome • Pregnancy-related hypertension • Pre-eclampsia • Eclampsia

KEY POINTS

- Preeclampsia is a multisystem disorder that can result in maternal morbidity and mortality.
- Preeclampsia usually manifests late in pregnancy with clinical manifestation of hypertension and proteinuria with or without edema.
- HELLP syndrome is a pregnancy-associated liver disease.
- Management of hypertension, seizure prevention, and planning for delivery are necessary to prevent HELLP syndrome.

INTRODUCTION/HISTORY/DEFINITIONS/BACKGROUND

Preeclampsia (PE) is the most common complication of pregnancy, and it occurs in approximately 5% of all pregnancies especially in middle and low-income countries.

PE is a multisystem disorder that can result in maternal morbidity and mortality, and usually manifests late in pregnancy.[1] PE was formerly referred to as toxemia and is diagnosed during pregnancy as the onset of hypertension and proteinuria with or without edema in legs, hands, and feet. PE is defined as being with or without severe features. Although PE can manifest early in pregnancy or immediately after delivery, it is most prevalent in the third trimester.

During pregnancy, the metabolic demand of the growing fetus causes physiologic changes in all body organs including the liver. However, a severe complication of PE is the HELLP syndrome. HELLP syndrome is a pregnancy-associated liver disease characterized by the presence of hemolysis (H), elevated liver enzymes, and low platelet count; however, these symptoms may or may not coexist with hypertension or proteinuria.[1]

"Hypertension is established with blood pressure greater than 140/90 mm Hg or mean arterial pressure greater than 105 mm Hg while proteinuria is the excretion of

[a] Louisiana State University Health New Orleans School of Nursing, The Louisiana Center for Promotion of Optimal Health Outcomes: A Joanna Briggs Institute,1900 Gravier Street, New Orleans, LA 70112, USA; [b] VP Quality Woman's Hospital, 100 Woman's Way, Baton Rouge, LA 70817, USA; [c] Adjunct Faculty Herzing University, 3900 North Causeway Blvd., Suite 800, Metairie, LA 70002, USA
* Corresponding author.
E-mail address: madorn@lsuhsc.edu

Crit Care Nurs Clin N Am 34 (2022) 277–288
https://doi.org/10.1016/j.cnc.2022.04.009
0899-5885/22/© 2022 Elsevier Inc. All rights reserved.
ccnursing.theclinics.com

30 mg/dL of protein in a random specimen ($\geq$1+ on urine dipstick) or 300 mg in a 24 h urine specimen."[1] Eclampsia is a complication of severe PE presenting with the new onset of grand mal seizure activity or coma with unknown etiology in a preeclamptic woman or occurring postpartum in a woman with signs or symptoms of PE. In most cases, about 80% of eclamptic seizures occur in the third trimester of pregnancy or within 48 hours postpartum. HELLP syndrome is considered a predisposing factor for the development of eclampsia.

In addition to defining blood pressure and proteinuria, PE with severe features is characterized by severe hypertension and $\leq$3+ of proteinuria or marginally reduced measurements (150/100 mm Hg and at least 2+ of proteinuria) coexisting with at least two symptoms of "imminent eclampsia".[2] Based on the onset of symptoms, PE can also be classified as early-onset preeclampsia (EOPE) occurring before 34 weeks of pregnancy, and late-onset preeclampsia, which manifests at week 34 of gestation or thereafter. Studies have shown a higher incidence of HELLP syndrome and eclampsia in EOPE.[1,3]

On an annual basis, as many as 500,000 mothers die as a result of pregnancy-related conditions mainly due to complications associated with PE, eclampsia and HELLP syndrome.[3] HELLP syndrome is a life-threatening condition and is the source of significant maternal and fetal risks and complications compounded by diagnostic and therapeutic issues.[4] The incidence of HELLP syndrome occurs in approximately 1 out of every 45,000 live births and complicates between 0.17% and 0.9% of all pregnancies.[3–8] In pregnancies complicated by PE with severe features, 10% to 30% of those women go on to develop HELLP syndrome.[2,4,6–8] In women who develop HELLP syndrome, serious complications occur in 12.5% and up to 65% of the cases.[9]

Pregnant and postpartum women are rarely admitted to the intensive care unit (ICU) and make up only 1% of all ICU admissions.[10] However, pregnancies complicated by the HELLP syndrome are a frequent cause of ICU admissions.[7] The complications of HELLP syndrome that may precipitate an ICU stay include placental abruption, acute kidney injury, hemolytic microangiopathic anemia, acute liver failure, liver capsule rupture, cerebral hemorrhage, cardiopulmonary compromise/failure, and disseminated intravascular coagulation (DIC).[7,11] HELLP syndrome is a progressive disease and severe complications and death are possible.[4]

Critical care of obstetric patients has received more attention recently with the previous focus primarily on maternity care, midwifery, and critical care practice.[12] A multidisciplinary team approach with care delivered in the ICU is ideal for women with HELLP syndrome.[13] Women with HELLP syndrome require intensive monitoring, prompt diagnosis, and treatment based on evidence-based protocols.[8,11] In most cases of HELLP syndrome, the intensive care nurse finds that there are two patients to assess and provide care.[14]

HELLP-ASSOCIATED MORBIDITY AND MORTALITY

Worldwide, hypertensive diseases of pregnancy are the leading cause of peripartum morbidity and mortality.[13] Maternal mortality due to HELLP syndrome is reported to be between 1% to 30%.[2,7] In 1% to 1.8% of the cases of HELLP syndrome, hepatic rupture occurs and is considered the most life-threatening complication of HELLP syndrome.[9] The hepatic rupture occurs most frequently in the anterior-superior region of the right hepatic lobe.[9]

Maternal mortality is most frequent when the mother's platelets are less than 50,000. This leads to DIC, which is present in approximately in 4% to 38% of HELLP syndrome cases.[11] However, DIC is not the primary symptom of HELLP but is a pathologic process of the disease that was not treated timely.[9] Most maternal deaths are associated with severe HELLP syndrome and is the result of delayed diagnosis, presence of infection, and renal failure.[15]

In autopsies performed on mothers who succumbed to the complications of HELLP, the findings included petechiae and suffusions in conjunctive tissue, skin and on mucous and serous surfaces of internal organs, cerebral edema, signs of acute respiratory distress syndrome (ARDS), edema of the lower extremities, hyperemia of the spleen, hydropericardium, and shock kidneys.[9] With HELLP syndrome, the significant postmortem finding are the liver findings including necrosis and hemorrhage.[9]

RISK FACTORS

Although HELLP syndrome presents suddenly and evades prediction, risk factors have been identified.[3] The risk factors for HELLP syndrome include multiparity and age over 30 years.[8] Conversely, nulliparity is a risk factor for hypertensive disorders of pregnancy.[16] Women with a previous history of HELLP syndrome and multiple gestation pregnancies are at risk.[16] White women of European descent are more likely to develop HELLP syndrome. Other risk factors include the following:

- Rural residence
- Pre-pregnancy hypertension
- Pre-pregnancy diabetes
- Gestational hypertension
- Chronic cardiac conditions
- Obesity
- Chronic hepatic conditions
- Placental disorders
- Congenital anomalies

Finally, there is reduced risk when there is premature rupture of the membranes and maternal age is less than 25 years.[17]

DIFFERENTIAL DIAGNOSIS AND CLINICAL PRESENTATION

There are multiple published classification systems for HELLP syndrome including the Mississippi and Tennessee taxonomies (**Table 1** HELLP Syndrome Classifications).[4,7,18] The Mississippi classification relies by the nadir platelet counts and the Tennessee classification is either complete or incomplete. The diagnosis of HELLP syndrome can be based solely on biochemical markers or a combination of symptoms and biochemical markers.[4]

The differential diagnosis of HELLP syndrome is complicated due to its presentation being similar to acute fatty liver of pregnancy (AFLP) and other liver diseases (**Table 2** Liver Diseases in Pregnancy).[2] Timely recognition and treatment of HELLP syndrome decreases maternal morbidity and mortality.[2] It has been estimated that there is a delay in the diagnosis by up to 8 days.[5] Incorrect diagnoses of HELLP syndrome include cholecystitis, esophagitis, gastritis, hepatitis, or idiopathic thrombocytopenia.[5]

Data from Corticelli A, Grimaldi M, Rosato BS, et al. Admission to intensive care unit for HELLP syndrome-9 years review in a low risk pregnant population. Gynecology & Obstetrics Care Report 2015; 1 (1:7): 1-2.

Differential diagnoses fall into four categories that include (a) diseases related to pregnancy, (b) infectious and inflammatory disease not related to pregnancy, (c) thrombocytopenia, and (d) rare diseases that resemble HELLP syndrome (**Table 3**

Table 1 HELLP syndrome classifications	
Class	**Description**
I	Platelet counts < 50,000 cells/µL
II	Platelet counts > 50,000 and < 100,000 cells/µL
III	Mild thrombocytopenia, Platelet nadir between > 100,000 and < 150,000 cells/µL
Mississippi Class I	Platelet counts < 50,000–100,000 cells/µL ALT or AST ≥ 70 LDH ≥ 600
Mississippi Class II	Platelet counts 50,000–100,000 cells/µL ALT or AST ≥ 70 LDH ≥ 600
Mississippi Class I	Platelet counts 100,000–150,000 cells/µL ALT or AST ≥ 40 LDH ≥ 600
Mississippi Partial	2 of 3 plus preeclampsia with severe features
Tennessee Complete HELLP	Platelet count < 100,00 AST > 70 LDH ≥ 600
Tennessee Partial HELLP	Meeting at least one criterion but not all

Abbreviations: AST, aspartate aminotransferase; LDH, Lactate dehydrogenase.

Data from Haram K, Svendsen E, Abildgaard U. The HELLP syndrome: Clinical issues and management. A review. BMC Pregnancy and Childbirth 2009; 9:8:1-15.; Poimenidi E, Metodiev Y, Archer NN, et al. Haemolysis, elevated liver enzymes and low platelets: Diagnosis and management in critical care 2021; 0:1-7.; Druzin ML, Shields LE, Peterson NL, et al. Preeclampsia toolkit: Improving health care response to preeclampsia (California Maternal Quality Care Collaborative Toolkit to Transform Maternity Care). Developed under contract #11-10006 with the California Department of Public Health; Maternal, Child and Adolescent Health Division; Published by the California Maternal Quality Care Collaborative, November 2013.

HELLP Syndrome Differential Diagnoses).[4] AFLP, thrombotic thrombocytopenic purpura, systemic lupus erythematosus, and hemolytic uremic syndrome represent some of the differential diagnoses for HELLP syndrome.[5]

The clinical progression of HELLP syndrome often includes a rapid deterioration of both maternal and fetal health requiring rapid identification and treatment.[3] Although the cause of HELLP syndrome is still not understood, the condition usually occurs between the 27th to the 37th week of pregnancy with 20% of the cases occurring in the postpartum period.[8] Women with HELLP syndrome present with general malaise, epigastric pain, headaches, and nausea and vomiting.[5] Tenderness in the right upper quadrant is present in about 90% of women with HELLP syndrome.[5] Edema is not a useful indicator as it is present in approximately 30% of pregnancies.[5]

For severe HELLP syndrome cases, oliguria may be present and is indicative of renal dysfunction.[16] Neurologic symptoms in HELLP include severe headaches (33%–61%) and visual disturbances (10%–20% of cases).[16] In the case of a delayed diagnosis of HELLP syndrome, DIC may present as the first noted clinical symptom.

Table 2
Liver diseases in pregnancy

Liver Disease	Trimester	Diagnostic Criteria
Hyperemesis gravidarum	1, 2	↑Bilirubin (× 2–4 ULN), ↑ALT/AST (× 2–4 ULN)
Intrahepatic cholestasis of pregnancy	1,2,3	↑Bilirubin (× 6 ULN), ↑ALT/AST (× 6 ULN), ↑Bile acids
Preeclampsia	2,3	↑Bilirubin (× 2–5 ULN), ↑ALT/AST (× 10–50 ULN), ↓platelets
HELLP syndrome	2,3	↑Bilirubin (× 10–20 ULN), ↑ LDH, ↓platelets, ↑ uric acid
Acute fatty liver of pregnancy	2,3	↑Bilirubin (× 6–8 ULN), ↑ALT/AST (× 5–10 ULN)—rarely>20

ALN: alanine aminotransferase, ALT: aspartate aminotransferase; ULN: upper limits of normal.

COMPLICATIONS OF HELLP SYNDROME

Although expectant management of HELLP syndrome is appropriate in many cases, women can also experience a rapid decline and the development of many morbidities.[10] Maternal morbidities are more serious when HELLP syndrome is of Class 1.[11] Additional morbidities include DIC, hepatic damage, acute kidney injury, placental abruption, preterm delivery, sepsis, ARDS, and stroke.[10,11,13] Acute kidney injury may result in the need for dialysis.[19]

A profound consequence of HELLP syndrome is acute liver failure.[4] One of the most fatal results of HELLP syndrome is the spontaneous subcapsular liver hematoma as it can result in exsanguination.[10] Toxins, poisoning, trauma and preexisting decompensating liver disease need to be excluded as a differential diagnosis of HELLP syndrome.[7] Acute liver failure can be exacerbated by viral hepatitis, Budd–Chiari syndrome and postpartum hemorrhage.[7]

When HELLP syndrome occurs in the postpartum period, maternal complications may include renal dysfunction and pulmonary edema.[10] Complications to the fetus include death, intrauterine growth retardation, respiratory distress syndrome, neonatal thrombocytopenia, and death.[4]

GUIDELINES FOR THERAPEUTIC TREATMENT OPTIONS

Management of HELLP syndrome includes monitoring of obstetric complications, management of hypertension, seizure prevention, and planning for delivery. Primary treatment is immediate delivery of the infant and placenta, regardless of gestation age at the time of diagnosis.[18] A management algorithm for HELLP syndrome can be found in **Table 4**.[20] Prompt vaginal or cesarean delivery is required due to the increased incidence of maternal morbidity and mortality and risk for patients to quickly deteriorate.[6,21] Determining the route of delivery should be based on the severity of the disease, maternal and infant status, and the likelihood of a successful induction of labor given the cervical status and obstetric history.[18] If the pregnancy is less than 34 weeks of gestation and the patient's status allows, the obstetrician may opt to delay delivery to allow for the administration of corticosteroids.[6,18,22,23]

The need for swift delivery, including in the case of preterm gestation, requires the involvement of a multidisciplinary team that is capable of providing intensive care to both the maternal and neonatal patient. Team members involved in the care of HELLP

Table 3 HELLP syndrome differential diagnoses	
Category	**Diagnosis**
Pregnancy-related conditions	Benign thrombocytopenia of pregnancy
	Acute fatty liver of pregnancy
Infectious and inflammatory diseases	Viral hepatitis
	Cholangitis
	Cholecystitis
	Upper respiratory tract infection
	Gastritis
	Gastric ulcer
	Acute pancreatitis
Thrombocytopenia	Immunologic thrombocytopenia
	Folate deficiency
	Systemic lupus erythematosus
	Antiphospholipid syndrome
Rare diseases that mimic HELLP syndrome	Thrombotic thrombocytopenic purpura
	Hemolytic uremic syndrome

Data from Haram K, Svendsen E, Abildgaard U. The HELLP syndrome: Clinical issues and management. A review. BMC Pregnancy and Childbirth 2009; 9:8:1-15.

syndrome patients should include the obstetric, perinatal, and neonatal teams, as well as a neonatal and adult intensive care team.[6,18] HELLP syndrome, in addition to PE with severe features and eclampsia, are all diagnoses that commonly lead to obstetric patients being admitted to the ICU. Admission to the ICU is recommended if there is need for ventilator support or if two or more organ systems start failing due to the increased risk of mortality for the patient and infant.[6,24]

ASSESSMENT OF LAB VALUES AND SYMPTOMS ASSOCIATED WITH HELLP

Close monitoring of the maternal laboratory values relevant to HELLP syndrome, including platelet count and liver enzymes, should be conducted at least every 12 hours throughout delivery and continue during the postpartum period. Typically, with HELLP syndrome liver enzyme levels will continue to increase as platelet levels continue to decrease even after delivery. The platelets are expected to reach their nadir on average 23 hours after birth, and the symptoms of HELLP syndrome are expected to peak within 2 days of delivery.[6] Additional assessments should be conducted as patients diagnosed with HELLP syndrome are at an increased risk of developing renal failure, ARDS, hemorrhage, and pulmonary edema.[6]

USE OF MAGNESIUM SULFATE AND ANTIHYPERTENSIVE MEDICATIONS IN THE TREATMENT OF

Administration of intravenous magnesium sulfate is recommended for pregnancies affected by HELLP syndrome or PE with severe features.[18] As a central nervous system depressant, magnesium sulfate has been found to be more effective at reducing the occurrence of eclampsia, recurrent seizures, and maternal death when compared with diazepam or phenytoin.[25–30] Magnesium sulfate should be administered with an initial loading dose over 15 to 20 minutes of 4 to 6 g followed by 1 to 2 g per hour maintenance dose. Patients whose body mass index is greater than 35 should be given a 6-g loading dose.[25,31,32]

Table 4
Management of HELLP syndrome

Gestational Age	Treatment
Any weeks' gestation	• Admit to labor and delivery or intensive care unit (pending severity of maternal symptoms) • IV magnesium sulfate • Antihypertensive if systolic blood pressure ≥160; or diastolic blood pressure ≥105 mm Hg
24–34 wk	• Refer to tertiary care facility • 24–48 h delay in delivery to allow for course of antenatal corticosteroids (pending patient stability)
<24 wk or >34 wk	• Immediate delivery

Data from Stella CL, Sibai BM. Preeclampsia: Diagnosis and management of the atypical presentation. The journal of maternal-fetal & neonatal medicine: the official journal of the European Association of Perinatal Medicine, the Federation of Asia and Oceania Perinatal Societies, the International Society of Perinatal Obstetricians. 2006;19(7):381-386. https://doi.org/10.1080/14767050600678337

Antihypertensive medications, in addition to magnesium sulfate, should be used to treat blood pressure values of ≥160 mm Hg systolic or ≥110 mm Hg diastolic.[25] Medications should be used to maintain blood pressures, with the goal of a systolic blood pressure between 140 and 150 mm Hg and a diastolic blood pressure between 90 and 100 mm Hg[25] with some guidelines suggesting lower goals of 130 to 150 systolic and 80 to 100 diastolic, respectively.[33] However, blood pressures should not drop below 15% to 25% of the patient's initial mean arterial pressure, due to the risk of decreased perfusion to the placenta and subsequent fetal distress from uteroplacental insufficiency.[25] Due to the possible comorbidities from untreated hypertension, antihypertensive therapy may also be considered for patients with blood pressures of greater than 155 systolic and greater than 105 diastolic (**Fig. 1.** Antihypertensive Treatment Algorithm for Hypertensive Emergencies).[18,25]

USE OF CORTICOSTEROIDS IN THE TREATMENT OF HELLP

Previous studies showed the possible benefit of corticosteroid therapy, particularly dexamethasone, in decreasing maternal mortality, reducing hospital stays, or delaying the onset of HELLP syndrome.[23,25,34–37] However, these previous studies were primarily observational or retrospective in design with limited participants and those finding were not confirmed in subsequent randomized control trials.[22,23,25,38]

The American College of Obstetricians and Gynecologists (ACOG) refers to a Cochrane Database Systematic Review which examined 11 randomized control trials of 550 women and showed that the use of antenatal or postpartum corticosteroids as a means of reducing the inflammatory response and improving the antepartum or postpartum course of HELLP syndrome was of no benefit in reducing maternal or infant mortality.[21] The sole benefit of the use of corticosteroids during the antepartum period was the increase in the mean platelet count, but increase was not of enough benefit to warrant inclusion in the standard treatment of HELLP syndrome.[39] However, the California Maternal Quality Care Collaborative does state that the use of corticosteroid therapy would still be justified in cases in which improvement in the patient's platelet count would be useful.[25]

Despite this evidence of limited benefit to the patient in the treatment of HELLP syndrome, ACOG does recommend the administration of corticosteroids for a planned

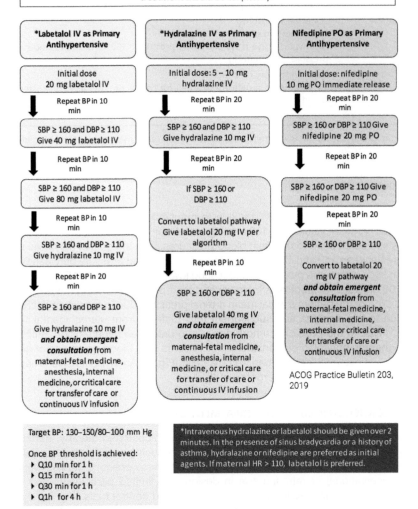

Treatment Recommendations for Sustained Systolic BP ≥ 160 mm Hg or Diastolic BP ≥ 110 mm Hg

*Antihypertensive treatment and magnesium sulfate should be administered simultaneously. If concurrent administration is not possible, antihypertensive treatment should be 1st priority.

*Labetalol IV as Primary Antihypertensive

Initial dose
20 mg labetalol IV
↓ Repeat BP in 10 min
SBP ≥ 160 and DBP ≥ 110 Give 40 mg labetalol IV
↓ Repeat BP in 10 min
SBP ≥ 160 and DBP ≥ 110 Give 80 mg labetalol IV
↓ Repeat BP in 10 min
SBP ≥ 160 and DBP ≥ 110 Give hydralazine 10 mg IV
↓ Repeat BP in 20 min
SBP ≥ 160 and DBP ≥ 110

Give hydralazine 10 mg IV *and obtain emergent consultation* from maternal-fetal medicine, anesthesia, internal medicine, or critical care for transfer of care or continuous IV infusion

*Hydralazine IV as Primary Antihypertensive

Initial dose: 5 – 10 mg hydralazine IV
↓ Repeat BP in 20 min
SBP ≥ 160 and DBP ≥ 110 Give hydralazine 10 mg IV
↓ Repeat BP in 20 min
If SBP ≥ 160 or DBP ≥ 110

Convert to labetalol pathway Give labetalol 20 mg IV per algorithm
↓ Repeat BP in 10 min
SBP ≥ 160 or DBP ≥ 110

Give labetalol 40 mg IV *and obtain emergent consultation* from maternal-fetal medicine, anesthesia, internal medicine, or critical care for transfer of care or continuous IV infusion

Nifedipine PO as Primary Antihypertensive

Initial dose: nifedipine 10 mg PO immediate release
↓ Repeat BP in 20 min
SBP ≥ 160 or DBP ≥ 110 Give nifedipine 20 mg PO
↓ Repeat BP in 20 min
SBP ≥ 160 or DBP ≥ 110 Give nifedipine 20 mg PO
↓ Repeat BP in 20 min
SBP ≥ 160 or DBP ≥ 110

Convert to labetalol 20 mg IV pathway *and obtain emergent consultation* from maternal-fetal medicine, internal medicine, anesthesia or critical care for transfer of care or continuous IV infusion

ACOG Practice Bulletin 203, 2019

Target BP: 130–150/80–100 mm Hg

Once BP threshold is achieved:
▸ Q10 min for 1 h
▸ Q15 min for 1 h
▸ Q30 min for 1 h
▸ Q1h for 4 h

*Intravenous hydralazine or labetalol should be given over 2 minutes. In the presence of sinus bradycardia or a history of asthma, hydralazine or nifedipine are preferred as initial agents. If maternal HR > 110, labetalol is preferred.

This figure was adapted from the Improving Health Care Response to Preeclampsia: A California Quality Improvement Toolkit, funded by the California Department of Public Health, 2014; supported by Title V funds.

Page 108

Fig. 1. is from the CMQCC Quality Improvement Toolkit which gives permission for reproduction. CMQCC-California Maternal Quality Care Collaborative. (This figure was adapted from the Improving Health Care Response to Preeclampsia: A California Quality Improvement Toolkit, funded by the California Department of Public Health, 2014; supported by Title V funds. Druzin M, Shields L, Peterson N, Sakowski C, Cape V, Morton C. Improving Health Care Response to Hypertensive Disorders of Pregnancy, a California Maternal Quality Care Collaborative Quality Improvement Toolkit, 2021. © 2021 California Maternal Quality Care Collaborative. The material in this toolkit may be freely reproduced and disseminated for informational, educational, and non-commercial purposes only. This toolkit was adapted from the Improving Health Care Response to Preeclampsia: A California Quality Improvement Toolkit, funded by the California Department of Public Health, 2014; supported by Title V funds.)

premature delivery before 34 weeks of gestation.[21] The administration of antenatal corticosteroids assists in enhancing fetal lung maturity and decrease the development of respiratory distress syndrome. Corticosteroids have also been found to decrease additional neonatal complications of premature birth including intraventricular hemorrhage and necrotizing enterocolitis.[25] If maternal and fetal status is stable and antenatal corticosteroids have not been administered in the last 2 weeks, then it may be appropriate to delay delivery for 24 to 48 hours to allow for the administration of corticosteroids.[6,18,22,23] The recommended dosage of corticosteroid therapy is two doses of 12 mg of Betamethasone or dexamethasone administered intramuscularly to the pregnant patient 12 to 24 hours apart depending on the need for quicker delivery.[25]

CARE CONSIDERATIONS FOR THE INTENSIVE CARE NURSE

The new mother who is diagnosed with HELLP syndrome may be admitted to the ICU while the newborn may be admitted to the neonatal intensive care unit (NICU). The critical care nurse will need to assist the new mother with postpartum care including both physical and emotional well-being. Postpartum care immediately following delivery should include fundal massage and lochia assessments every 15 minutes. Given the increased risk of postpartum hemorrhage, perineal pads should be weighed to obtain quantified blood loss amounts.

After patient stabilization, nursing interventions should focus on assistance with bonding and maternal role attainment. If the patient wishes to breastfeed, the hospital's lactation consultants should be notified, and the patient should be set up on a breast pump ideally within 6 hours of birth. If patient status allows, assisting with skin-to-skin contact with the infant or if the baby was born premature, allowing them to visit and view the baby in the NICU can help promote bonding. Health care providers must recognize the emotional, financial, and social implications associated with a maternal illness and an infant who may be admitted to the NICU.[40]

IMPLICATIONS FOR RESEARCH

According to the National Institute of Health (NIH), several researchers have reported that genetic factors in both the mother and the fetus can cause the development of PE and HELLP syndrome. Research findings also support that genetic and environmental factors interact, yet there is no one gene responsible for HELLP. Some women may have risk factors, but they may never develop HELLP syndrome. Although the cause of HELLP syndrome is not known, it is most common in women with PE or eclampsia.

Several risk factors such as liver biomarkers can predict the occurrence and outcomes of PE.[1,41]

SUMMARY

The exact causes of HELLP syndrome are still unknown; however, the importance of early diagnosis and supportive interventions can assist with ensuring the well-being of both the mother and the baby; thereby decreasing mortality and morbidity. The management of HELLP syndrome includes monitoring of obstetric complications, controlling of hypertension, seizure prevention, and planning for delivery. The primary treatment is the immediate delivery of the infant and placenta, regardless of gestation age at the time of diagnosis.[18] However, prematurely born infants may have multiple complications; therefore delivery may be delayed for pregnancies less than 34 weeks of gestation to allow for the administration of corticosteroids.[6,18,22,23] Managing

HELLP syndrome involves thorough assessment and prompt treatment of the patient to ensure a safe delivery of the infant and decrease postpartum complications for the mother. Women with HELLP syndrome require intensive monitoring, prompt diagnosis, and treatment according to evidence-based protocols.

CLINICS CARE POINTS

- Primary treatment is the immediate delivery of the infant and placenta.
- Delivery may be delayed if the pregnancy is less than 34 weeks of gestation to allow for the administration of corticosteroids.
- Admission to the intensive care unit (ICU) is recommended if there is need for ventilator support or if two or more organ systems start failing.
- Nursing interventions must facilitate bonding for the mother and the infant in the ICU.
- Magnesium sulfate is more effective at reducing the occurrence of eclampsia, recurrent seizures, and maternal death when compared with diazepam or phenytoin.
- Antihypertensive medications, in addition to magnesium sulfate, should be used to treat blood pressure values of $\geq$160 mm Hg systolic or $\geq$110 mm Hg diastolic.
- Women with HELLP syndrome require intensive monitoring, prompt diagnosis, and treatment according to evidence-based protocols.

DISCLOSURE

Author has nothing to disclose.

REFERENCES

1. Alese MO, Modley J, Naicker T. Preeclampsia and HELLP syndrome, the role of the liver. J Maternal-Fetal Neonatal Med 2021;34(1):117–23.
2. Alev AA, Hatice I, Zuhat A, et al. Factors determining the intensive care need in HELLP syndrome & AFLP in pregnancy. J Reprod Gynaecolgy Obstet 2021. Available at: https://www.heraldopenaccess.us/openaccess/factors-determining-the-intensive-care-need-in-help-syndrome-aflp-in-pregnancy. Accessed August 30, 2021.
3. Gedik E, Neslihan Y, Sahin T, et al. Hemolysis, elevated liver enzymes and low platelet syndrome: outcomes for patients admitted to intensive care at a tertiary referral hospital. Hypertens Pregnancy 2017;36(1):21–9.
4. Haram K, Svendsen E, Abildgaard U. The HELLP syndrome: clinical issues and management. A review. BMC Pregnancy and Childbirth 2009;9(8):1–15.
5. Padden MO. HELLP syndrome: recognition and perinatal management. Am Fam Physician 1999;60(3):829–36.
6. Lam MT, Dierking E. Intensive care unit issues in eclampsia and HELLP syndrome. Int J Crit Illness Inj Sci 2017;7(3):136–41.
7. Poimenidi E, Metodiev Y, Archer NN, et al. Haemolysis, elevated liver enzymes and low platelets: diagnosis and management in critical care. Journal of Intensive Care Society 2021;0:1–7.
8. Corticelli A, Grimaldi M, Rosato BS, et al. Admission to intensive care unit for HELLP syndrome-9 years review in a low risk pregnant population. Gynecol Obstet Care Rep 2015;1(1:7):1–2.

9. Tsokos M. Pathological features of maternal death from HELLP syndrome. In: Tsokos M, editor. Forensic pathology reviews volume 1. Forensic pathology reviews, Humana Press, Totowa (NJ). https://doi.org/10.1007/978-1-59259-786-4_12.

10. Kelsey JJ. Obstetric emergencies in the ICU. Critical and urgent care 2006. Available at: https://www.accp.com/docs/bookstore/psap/p7b02sample01.pdf. Accessed August 30, 2021.

11. Rojas-Suarez J, Vigil-De Gracia P. Pre-eclampsia eclampsia admitted to critical care unit. J Matern Fetal Neonatal Med 2012;25(10):2051–4.

12. Hinton L, Locock L, Knight M. Maternal critical care: what can we learn from patient experience? A qualitative study. BMJ Open 2015;5:1–9.

13. Arulkumaran N, Lightstone L. Severe pre-eclampsia and hypertensive crises. Best Pract Res Clin Obstet Gynaecol 2013;27:877–84.

14. Guntapalli KK, Hall N, Karnad DR, et al. Critical illness in pregnancy. Part 1: an approach to a pregnant patient in the ICU and common obstetric disorders. Contemp Rev Crit Care Med 2015;148(4):1093–104.

15. Eser B, Guven M, Unal A, et al. The role of plasma exchange in HELLP syndrome. Clin Appl Thrombosis/hemostasis 2005;11(2):211–7.

16. Rath W, Tsikouras P, Stelzl P. HELLP syndrome or acute fatty liver of pregnancy: a differential diagnostic challenge. Geburtsh Frauenheilk 2020;80:499–507.

17. What are the key risk factors for HELLP syndrome: in: ObG Project Grand Rounds. Available at: https://www.obgproject.com/2020/06/10/what-are-the-key-risk-factors-for-hellp-syndrome/. Accessed September 3, 2021.

18. Druzin ML, Shields LE, Peterson NL, et al. Preeclampsia toolkit: Improving health care response to preeclampsia (California Maternal Quality Care Collaborative Toolkit to Transform Maternity Care). Developed under contract #11-10006 with the California Department of Public Health; Maternal, Child and Adolescent Health Division; Published by the California Maternal Quality Care Collaborative, 2013.

19. Erlangga ME, Pradian E, Sudjud RW et al. Case report: intensive care management of preeclampsia and HELLP syndrome. J Health Med Sci; 3(3): 370-392.

20. Stella CL, Sibai BM. Preeclampsia: diagnosis and management of the atypical presentation. J Matern Fetal Neonatal Med 2006;19(7):381–6.

21. Hypertension in pregnancy. Report of the American College of Obstetricians and Gynecologists' Task Force on Hypertension in Pregnancy. Obstetrics and Gynecology 2013;122(5):1122-31. doi:10.1097/01.AOG.0000437382.03963.88.

22. ACOG. Hypertension in Pregnancy: report of the American College of obstetricians and Gynecologists' task force on hypertension in pregnancy. Obstet Gynecol 2013;122(5):1122–31.

23. Sibai BM, Stella CL. Diagnosis and management of atypical preeclampsia-eclampsia. Am J Obstet Gynecol 2009;200(5):481.e1-7.

24. Trikha A, Singh P. The critically ill obstetric patient – recent concepts. Indian J Anaesth 2010;54:421–7.

25. Druzin M, Shields L, Peterson N, et al. Improving Health Care Response to Hypertensive Disorders of Pregnancy, a California Maternal Quality Care Collaborative Quality Improvement Toolkit, 2021.

26. Altman D, Carroli G, Duley L, et al. Do women with pre-eclampsia, and their babies, benefit from magnesium sulphate? The Magpie Trial: a randomized placebo-controlled trial. Lancet 2002;359:1877–90.

27. Duley L, Gulmezoglu AM, Chou D. Magnesium sulphate versus lytic cocktail for eclampsia. Cochrane Database Syst Rev 2010:CD002960. https://doi.org/10.1002/14651858.CD002960.pub2.

28. Duley L, Henderson-Smart D. Magnesium sulphate versus phenytoin for eclampsia. Cochrane Database Syst Rev 2003:CD000128. https://doi.org/10.1002/14651858.CD000128.

29. Duley L, Matar HE, Almerie MQ, et al. Alternative magnesium sulphate regimens for women with preeclampsia and eclampsia. Cochrane Database Syst Rev 2010:CD007388. https://doi.org/10.1002/14651858.CD007388.pub2.

30. Coetzee EJ, Dommisse J, Anthony J. A randomised controlled trial of intravenous magnesium sulphate versus placebo in the management of women with severe pre-eclampsia. Br J Obstet Gynaecol 1998;105:300–3.

31. Brookfield KF, Elkomy M, Su F, et al. Optimization of maternal magnesium sulfate administration for fetal neuroprotection: application of a prospectively constructed pharmacokinetic model to the BEAM cohort. J Clin Pharmacol 2017; 57:1419–24.

32. Dayicioglu V, Sahinoglu Z, Kol E, et al. The use of standard dose of magnesium sulphate in prophylaxis of eclamptic seizures: do body mass index alterations have any effect on success? Hypertens Pregnancy 2003;22:257–65.

33. World Health Organization. WHO recommendations for prevention and treatment of pre-eclampsia and eclampsia. 2011. Available at: https://www.who.int/reproductivehealth/publications/maternal_perinatal_health/9789241548335/en/. Accessed February 9, 2022.

34. HELLP syndrome. Preeclampsia foundation. Available at: https://www.preeclampsia.org/hellp-syndrome. Accessed August 27, 2021.

35. Haddad B, Deis S, Goffinet F, et al. Maternal and perinatal outcomes during expectant management of 239 severe preeclamptic women between 24 and 33 weeks' gestation. Am J Obstet Gynecol 2004;190:1590–5 [discussion: 1595-1597].

36. Sibai B, Ramadan M, Usta I, et al. Maternal morbidity and mortality in 442 pregnancies with hemolysis, elevated liver enzymes, and low platelets (HELLP Syndrome). Am J Obstet Gynecol 1993;169:1000–6.

37. Martin J, Brewer J, Wallace K, et al. HELLP Syndrome and composite major maternal morbidity: importance of Mississippi classification system. Matern Fetal Neonatal Med 2013. https://doi.org/10.3109/14767058.2013.773308. Epub ahead of print.

38. Martin JN Jr, Brewer JM, Wallace K, et al. HELLP syndrome and composite major maternal morbidity: importance of Mississippi classification system. J Matern Fetal Neonatal Med 2013;26:1201–6.

39. Woudstra DM, Chandra S, Hofmeyr GJ, et al. Corticosteroids for HELLP (hemolysis, elevated liver enzymes, low platelets) syndrome in pregnancy. Cochrane Database Syst Rev 2010;9:1–73. Art. No.: CD008148. (Systematic Review and Meta-Analysis).

40. Barnhart L. HELLP syndrome and the effects on the neonate. Neonatal Netw 2015;34(5):1–5.

41. National Institutes of Health (NIH). Available at: https://rarediseases.info.nih.gov/diseases/8528/hellp-syndrome. Accessed February 1, 2022.

Hepatocellular Carcinoma

HoChong Gilles, DNP, FNP-BC, AF-AASLD*, Tonora Garbutt, DNP, RN, NEA-BC,
Jasmine Landrum, DNP, RN

KEYWORDS

- Hepatocellular carcinoma • Cirrhosis • Surgical resection • Liver transplantation
- Thermal ablation • Intraarterial therapy • Systemic therapy

KEY POINTS

- Hepatocellular carcinoma (HCC) is a primary liver malignancy arising from underlying chronic liver disease and cirrhosis.
- Imaging plays an important role in HCC diagnosis. LIRADS provides a standardized method of reporting liver observations to guide treatment options.
- Staging systems are useful in predicting prognosis and advise therapeutic strategies. The Barcelona Clinic Liver Cancer staging system is commonly used to stratify patients based on tumor size, number of liver lesions, liver function, and performance status.
- Curative options for HCC include surgical resection, liver transplantation, and thermal ablation.
- Noncurative options include intraarterial therapy, radiation, and systemic therapy. Each modality is aimed to slow the progression of disease and improve overall survival.

Hepatocellular carcinoma (HCC) is a primary liver malignancy commonly encountered in the setting of chronic liver disease and cirrhosis.[1] In the past 2 decades, the incidence of HCC has dramatically risen and ranks as the 5th most common malignancy reported by the World Health Organization and a leading cause of cancer-related mortality in the United States.[2] Advances in curative and noncurative options have improved treatment response and overall survival. Management of HCC is complex, and choice of treatment is enhanced by multidisciplinary consensus, including a liver transplant center.

The major risk factor associated with HCC is chronic liver injury resulting from any etiology that progresses to cirrhosis. Globally, hepatitis B virus (HBV) and hepatitis C virus (HCV) are the main causal agents of cirrhosis and the incidence rate of HCC development in patients with established cirrhosis is approximately 2% to 4% per year.[3] Due to improved HBV vaccination rates and highly effective antiviral agents for HCV, the incidence of cirrhosis from viral hepatitis is projected to decline over the years. However, due to the high prevalence of nonalcoholic fatty liver disease (NAFLD) and alcohol-associated liver disease (ALD) in the US, cirrhosis secondary

Central Virginia Veterans Affairs Medical Center, 1201 Broad Rock Blvd (111N), Richmond, VA 23249, USA
* Corresponding author.
E-mail address: Hochong.gilles@va.gov

to NAFLD and ALD will become major contributors to the development of HCC.[4] In most countries, HCC rates are 2 to 4 times higher in men compared with women.[2] However, females are at a higher median age at the time of HCC diagnosis. According to race, American Indian/Alaskan Natives and Hispanics have the highest incidence of HCC in the US.[5]

PROGNOSIS IN HEPATOCELLULAR CARCINOMA

HCC is considered different from other primary malignancies as its prognosis is also dependent on underlying liver function plus tumor staging and performance status.[6] Available treatment modalities can be limited in the setting of poor liver function. Treatment outcomes in HCC are determined by the ABCs: anatomy, biologic grade, and cirrhosis severity. **Table 1**.

Survival outcomes in HCC vary by etiology but are considered poor overall. The 5-year survival is estimated at less than 20% as patients are often diagnosed with advanced-stage disease at the initial time of diagnosis.[7] Additionally, patients with advanced cirrhosis often die from liver failure rather than the progression of their cancer.

PROGNOSIS IN CIRRHOSIS

The Child-Pugh (CP) score and Model for End-Stage Liver Disease (MELD) are common scoring systems used in the clinic practice to assess the prognosis and severity of cirrhosis. Originally, the Child-Turcotte score was first introduced back in 1964 to predict mortality after portal decompression surgery.[8] The score was modified, substituting the prothrombin time for nutrition status and later became known as the CP score.[9,10] The CP score is determined by 5 factors: total bilirubin level, serum albumin, prothrombin time, ascites, and hepatic encephalopathy. The CP score depends on the clinical assessment of ascites and encephalopathy, which may result in variation in scoring among providers.

Table 1
HCC outcome factors

	Favorable Outcome	Poor Outcome
Anatomy (stage)		
Size and number of lesions	Small and solitary	Large and multi-focal
Nodal or extrahepatic metastases	Absent	Present
Biological aggressiveness (grade)		
Histologic feature	Well differentiated	Poorly differentiated
Vascular invasion	Absent	Present
Growth/metabolic rate	Slow	Rapid
Cirrhosis Severity		
	Compensated	Decompensated
	Child-Pugh A	Child-Pugh B-C
ECOG Performance Status		
	PS 0	PS 3–4

Abbreviation: ECOG, eastern cooperative oncology group.
Data from Brar G, Greten TF, Graubard BI, et al. Hepatocellular Carcinoma Survival by Etiology: A SEER-Medicare Database Analysis. Hepatol Commun. 2020;4(10):1541-1551. Published 2020 Aug 9. https://doi.org/10.1002/hep4.1564; and Duseja, Ajay. "Staging of hepatocellular carcinoma." Journal of clinical and experimental hepatology. 2014; 4: S74-S79.

CP Class A: 5–6 points.

- Least severe liver disease
- One- to 5-year survival rate: 95%[9,10]

CP Class B: 7 to 9 points.

- Moderately severe liver disease
- One- to 5-year survival rate: 75%[9,10]

CP Class C: 10–15 points.

- Most severe liver disease
- One- to 5-year survival rate: 50%[9,10]

The MELD score was derived by multivariate analysis of predictors of 90-day mortality in patients with cirrhosis undergoing transjugular intrahepatic portosystemic shunt.[11] The MELD score consists of 3 laboratory parameters including the international normalized ratio (INR), bilirubin, and serum creatinine. Although there are limitations in this calculation, the MELD score can predict end-stage liver disease and median survival at 3 months.[12] Since 2002, the organ allocation for liver transplant in the US has been based on the MELD score. The MELD score range is 6–40 points. The higher the score, the higher the 3-month mortality related to their liver disease. The MELD- Na became the new standard for organ allocation for liver transplantation in January 2016 due to improved prediction of pretransplant mortality. However, the MELD score does not always accurately predict survival in all patients with cirrhosis. Conditions such as liver cancer are associated with a higher mortality rate than the MELD score would reflect and therefore, receive additional MELD points when listed for liver transplantation.

DIAGNOSIS OF HEPATOCELLULAR CARCINOMA

HCC is typically an asymptomatic disease. Diagnosis of HCC based on symptoms is rare unless patients present with advanced or late-stage disease. Therefore, imaging plays a significant role in making the radiologic diagnosis of HCC. Early detection of small tumors in the background of a cirrhotic liver remains challenging.[13] However, improvement of imaging techniques permits clinicians to accurately characterize and diagnose HCC without biopsy confirmation. Multi-phase CT or MRI is the preferred imaging modality when there is a suspicion of HCC or abnormal findings revealed on a screening ultrasound.[1] Features of enhancement patterns compared with the background liver are important in the arterial, portal venous, and later phases.[14] Imaging appearances vary between HCC and the cirrhotic liver. These hallmark differences include arterial phase nonrim hyperenhancement, portal venous washout relative to the background liver, and capsule rim enhancement permit reliable radiologic characterization of HCC in lesions >/ = to 2 cm.[15,16]

Previously, there was no standardized reporting of imaging before the American College of Radiology publishing a guideline on how CT/MRI images should be performed, interpreted, and reported until 2011. The Liver Imaging Reporting and Data System (LIRADS) provide a consistent framework for reporting liver lesions to help determine surveillance and treatment options.[17] Application of LIRADS only applies to patients at risk for HCC:

- Cirrhosis of any etiology
- Chronic Hepatitis B infection
- Current or prior history of HCC

LIRADS (LR) categories are defined as:

- LR 1: Definitely benign
- LR 2: Probably benign
- LR 3: Intermediate for malignancy
- LR 4: Probable HCC
- LR 5: Definitely HCC
  - Lesions >/ = 2 cm require arterial phase enhancement and 1 of the following:
    - Washout
    - Capsule enhancement
    - Threshold growth
  - Lesions 10 to 19 mm require 2 of the following
    - Washout
    - Capsule enhancement
    - Threshold growth
- LR M: Probably/definite malignancy but not necessarily HCC
- LR-TIV: Tumor in veins

Data from CT/MRI LI-RADS v2018 CORE accessed at https://www.acr.org/Clinical-Resources/Reporting-and-Data-Systems/LI-RADS/CT-MRI-LI-RADS-v2018

LIRADS 5 lesions provide a radiologic diagnosis of HCC and are easily adapted to the Organ Procurement and Transplantation Network (OPTN) class 5 criteria needed to obtain a MELD exception score for liver transplantation prioritization.[1,3] The role of liver biopsy should be considered if the liver lesion observation does not have typical enhancement patterns for definitive HCC or appearance is suggestive of other malignancy.

STAGING

Staging systems are useful in predicting prognosis and guiding therapeutic options.[18] There are various validated staging systems for HCC. A system implemented by the American Joint Commission on Cancer is the tumor/node/metastasis (TNM) classification system. This anatomic staging system accounts for tumor characteristics which include tumor size, number of lesions, and presence of vascular invasion, in addition to lymph node involvement and metastatic disease.[19] The TNM staging is mainly used when examining tissue obtained during surgical resection.

In addition to the TNM staging system for HCC, other systems have been proposed to help guide therapeutic strategies. The Barcelona Clinic Liver Cancer (BCLC) staging system is a validated staging and treatment system that stratifies patients based on tumor size, number of lesions, underlying liver function, and performance status.[20] The BCLC staging system is often thought to be superior to other staging systems in determining prognosis given the inclusion of liver function and performance status. However, a one-size-fits-all staging system has not been universally adopted. **Table 2**.

CURATIVE OPTIONS

Advances in surgical and therapeutic options have improved treatment response and survival. Surgical resection, liver transplant, and thermal ablation in selected patients can potentially cure HCC leading to improved survival.

Surgical Resection

Surgical resection is favored and recommended for patients with a solitary liver mass without cirrhosis or cirrhosis with preserved liver function (BCLC Stage 0).[21]

Table 2
Barcelona staging and treatment algorithm

Stage	Size/Number of lesions	Child-Pugh	Performance Status	LT Candidacy	Treatment Option
Very early (0)	Solitary <2 cm	A	0	No	Ablation
Early (A)	Single up to 3 lesions < 3 cm	A-B	0	Yes with no PHTN Yes with PHTN No	Resection Transplant Ablation
Intermediate (B)	Large and multifocal	A-B	0		Intraarteria
Advanced (C)	Portal invasion Extrahepatic spread	A-B	1–2		Systemic
Terminal (D)		C	3–4		Standard of Care

Data from Llovet JM, Di Bisceglie AM, Bruix J, et al. Design and endpoints of clinical trials in hepatocellular carcinoma. J Natl Cancer Inst. 2008;100(10):698-711. https://doi.org/10.1093/jnci/djn134.

Unfortunately, most of the patients have cirrhosis, and the ability to tolerate curative resection may be limited. The extent of resection (anatomic wedge vs segmentectomy vs hepatectomy) is dependent on liver function, absence of clinically significant portal hypertension, and remaining liver volume. 5-year survival after resection is approximately 74% in patients without portal hypertension but drops to approximately 50% to 60% when clinically relevant portal hypertension is present.[20] Surgical resection using a minimally invasive laparoscopic approach has similar survival outcomes to open resection and may offer additional benefits, including decreased postoperative complications and shorter length of stay.[22] The risk of recurrence after resection is approximately 70% within 5 years.[23] Recurrence can be either new or residual liver cancer. Important pathologic predictors for recurrence include positive surgical margins, advanced tumor grade, micro and macrovascular invasion, and presence of satellite nodules. However, long-term survival can be achieved after successful surgical resection in select populations.

Liver Transplantation

Liver transplantation is considered an effective therapy for early-stage HCC (BCLC Stage 0-A) in patients otherwise considered a candidate for transplant.[1] Transplant is often considered superior to resection because it offers treatment of both HCC and underlying cirrhosis. Liver transplant is the only surgical procedure that can reverse portal hypertension and is associated with a 5-year survival of approximately 70% for HCC transplanted within the Milan criteria.[24] Early experience in liver transplantation for HCC before the Milan criteria achieved unacceptable long-term outcomes with half the deaths resulting from tumor recurrence. The Milan criteria define a solitary lesion measuring 2 to 5 cm or up to 3 lesions, all measuring < 3 cm, without evidence of extrahepatic spread. This pivotal study conducted by Mazzaferro and colleagues demonstrated that patients within this criterion had improved disease-free survival at 4 years, which led to a renewed enthusiasm for liver transplant for HCC. Due to limited organ availability, the United Network of Organ Sharing (UNOS) adopted the Milan criteria in considering patients with HCC for liver transplant under a standardized MELD exception. If a patient's calculated MELD score does not reflect their disease severity or medical urgency for liver transplant, UNOS permits a liver transplant center to request a MELD exception score.

Subsequent studies found that some candidates beyond the Milan criteria could be transplanted successfully. This approach is termed "downstaging." Stage III tumors (beyond Milan criteria) would undergo locoregional therapy and follow-up imaging showing control and absence of progression could be reclassified as "down-staged" within Milan and therefore, considered for liver transplant also under MELD exception. Studies showed success in downstaging selected patients with favorable tumor grade achieved excellent posttransplant survival.[25] Additionally, due to anticipated waiting times for organ availability, various locoregional therapies can be used as a bridge therapy to prevent disease progression and reduce wait list removal.[26] The key concept in using locoregional therapy in downstaging and minimizing wait list progression is to allow the distinction of indolent from aggressive forms of HCC to improve wait list and posttransplant outcomes.

Thermal Ablation

Ablation therapy is a medical treatment modality that destroys abnormal tissue cells through the use of chemical, heat, and cold applications. Ablation therapy is considered a preferred treatment option for BCLC Stage 0-A tumors, otherwise not suitable for surgical intervention. The percutaneous approach for ablation therapy uses a specialized needle, which is passed from the skin directly into the tumor with minimal invasiveness. The most common types of ablation therapy used to treat patients with HCC are ethanol injection, radiofrequency ablation, microwave ablation, and cryoablation.

Percutaneous Ethanol Injection (PEI) is a form of chemical ablation therapy using 95%–100% ethanol alcohol injected into the hepatic tumor. PEI was the first ablative technique used for HCC. However, current health care technological advances have paved the way for other ablative techniques requiring less treatment frequency and yielding superior outcomes.[27] Radiofrequency ablation (RFA) is used to treat HCC percutaneously or laparoscopically. RFA uses high-frequency alternating energy, which is converted to heat from the exposed tip of the electrode.[28] This controlled application of heat destroys the malignant tissue and reduces the tumor size by necrosis. RFA is known to be superior to PEI in nodules between 2 and 4 cm.[29] Limitations of RFA include the heat sink effect that can decrease its efficacy especially in larger tumors and inability to treat in difficult locations, especially near the biliary tree or other vital organs.

Microwave ablation (MWA) destroys tumor tissue by direct hyperthermic injury produced by electromagnetic waves emitted from the noninsulated portions of the antenna. MWA can be considered to have advantages over RFA for its shorter procedure times, greater yield of active heating, and decreased risk of incomplete ablation.[29] MWA may be able to treat larger tumors more effectively and have less concerns for heat sinks. Cryoablation is an alternative to the heat-based ablative techniques, which uses the extreme subzero cold application to destroy hepatic tumors by freezing tissue between −20 and 60° Celsius. Cryoablation paired with imaging modalities provides optimal control of treatment monitoring and effects.[29] Different types of ablation depend on the availability of local expertise and resources.

The benefits of ablation therapy are cost, candidacy, and recovery. Percutaneous ablation can be performed in an outpatient setting reducing the need for hospital admission. Patients who are not good candidates for general anesthesia can undergo ablation therapy using conscious sedation or monitored anesthesia care. Recovery time is shorter resulting in the patient going home the same day of the procedure, or in some cases only requiring an observation stay.

NONCURATIVE OPTIONS

Noncurative approaches include intraarterial, radiation, and systemic therapies which aim to palliate or slow the progression of disease.

INTRAARTERIAL/LOCOREGIONAL THERAPIES
Transarterial Chemoembolization

Transarterial chemoembolization (TACE) is the standard treatment of intermediate-BCLC stage B HCC. TACE allows selective delivery of a chemotherapeutic agent to hepatic tumors and protects against ischemic necrosis to the rest of the liver.[30] There are diverse treatment modalities using TACE or combination therapy in patients with early, intermediate, or advanced HCC.[31] TACE is the umbrella term to describe several fundamentally different procedures including conventional TACE methods, TACE with drug-eluting beads, and transarterial embolization (TAE).[32] Transarterial Embolization (TAE) is very similar to TACE except no chemotherapeutic agent is used. The lesion is treated with simple particle embolization. Conventional TACE (cTACE) uses Lipiodol, as an embolic material vigorously mixed with various anticancer drugs.[31] Doxorubicin is the most commonly used cytotoxic agent. Lipiodol acts as a micro-vessel embolic agent and has antitumor effects by impeding blood flow, thereby increasing chemotherapeutic distribution.[32]

Transarterial Chemoembolization with Drug-Eluting Beads

Experts recommend the combination of drug-eluting beads (DEB) and TACE to sequester chemotherapeutic agents into the systemic circulation and sharply increase the local drug concentration. As an alternative to cTACE, DEB-TACE was developed to release the cytotoxic drug doxorubicin in a sustained manner in the form of nonresorbable microspheres. DEB-TACE has demonstrated a significant reduction in liver toxicity and drug-related adverse events. In terms of clinical efficacy, no prospective study has reported a significant difference among cTACE and DEB-TACE.[31]

Combination Therapy with Transarterial Chemoembolization

Tumor recurrence after TACE is common and repeat TACE might worsen liver function and adversely affect patient survival. Therefore, a combination strategy with ablation treatment can provide better local control of disease than TACE alone in patients with intermediate or large HCC.[30,31] TACE combined with ablation attained better survival rates at the 1-, 2-, 3- and 5-year marks.[31] Therefore, TACE combined with RFA is a safe and effective treatment strategy for patients with intermediate-stage HCC.

Transarterial Chemoembolization Nursing Implications

Navigating the various HCC treatment therapies, experiences, and symptom management can be challenging for nurses. It is not always easy to determine whether the source of symptoms is caused by illness or treatment. Starting treatment provides a sense of control over the disease and offers a way to cope with the diagnosis. However, treatment-related adverse events can be perceived as symptoms of HCC and liver failure, making patients uncertain about the effect of treatment versus worsening HCC.[33]

    A common clinical manifestation is postchemoembolization syndrome caused by TACE. Chemoembolization syndrome can further reflect the degree of tumor necrosis and the effectiveness of embolization.[34] This occurrence may be related to the complete vascular embolization of the tumor, necrosis, or the size/strength of the DEB-TACE.[35] After sufficient tumor necrosis, patients are prone to fever, pain, nausea, and vomiting induced by embolization and tumor necrosis.[34] Through predictive nursing, nurses can strengthen patient education of adverse events, incorporate psychological nursing, and provide supportive care throughout the effects of treatment.

Transarterial Radioembolization

Transarterial radioembolization (TARE) is a minimally invasive intraarterial therapy that delivers radioactive microbeads containing B-emitting Yttrium-90 isotopes directly into the tumor via hepatic artery branches.[36] TARE is also known as a selective internal radiation therapy. TARE disrupts the pathophysiology of HCC by changing the perfusion pattern to allow tumoricidal doses of radiation to be locally administered. This method spares healthy liver and has minimal toxicity risk to the patient. The TARE treatment modality offers the benefit of slowing the disease progression and prolonging survival for patients with advanced or unresectable disease. TARE has given promising results in intermediate and advanced-stage HCC with disease control and an adequate tolerability profile.[37] Preselection of a TARE candidate requires diagnostic angiography called "mapping." The angiography aims to evaluate vascular anatomy and identify any extrahepatic branch which could disperse the microspheres to nontargeted organs, especially the lungs.[37] When comparing TACE and radioembolization, studies have shown that the median time to progression was longer after radioembolization and was associated with a more favorable safety profile.[37] TheraSphere and Sir-Spheres are commercially available options for TARE treatment.

Transarterial Radioembolization Nursing Implications

Complications typically occur due to a toxic dose administered to nontumoral tissues, or by procedural complications during the catheter's placement and manipulation.[37] Complications include:

- Liver failure or radio-induced liver disease (RILD) (4%)
- Biliary complication (<10%)
- Postradioembolization syndrome (PRS) (20%-55%)
- Fatigue
- Nausea
- Vomiting
- Anorexia
- Fever
- Abdominal pain
- Gastrointestinal complications (<5%)
- Radio-induced pneumonia (<1%)

The mapping selection phase is crucial to reduce the likelihood of these complications. The use of pretreatment medications can also help ameliorate symptoms. To achieve favorable outcomes, nurses and other health care providers must be aware of complications associated with TARE and consider pretreatment medications to decrease the likelihood of complications.

Stereotactic Body Radiation Therapy

Stereotactic body radiation therapy (SBRT) was introduced as a palliative treatment of unresectable HCC. Traditional radiation therapy had limited application in HCC because of the radiosensitivity of hepatocytes. SBRT focuses high energy on the target with better sparing of the surrounding tissue.[38] Before treatment, fiducial markers are placed near the tumor, treatment plan is mapped and administered in interval sessions. A large study reported 1-year survival of 81% and 2-year survival of 56% with local control of 99% at 2 years.[39] However, additional data are required for the inclusion of SBRT in management guidelines for HCC. The role of SBRT has expanded and is often used when other locoregional therapy is not feasible or as a bridge to liver transplantation.[40]

Pros[38,39]
- Focal, limit radiation-induced liver injury
- Administered efficiently on an outpatient basis
- Well tolerated
- No sedation

Cons[38,39]
- Acute and long-term toxicity, including radiation-induced liver damage
- Less efficacy in larger tumors
- Motion management
- Dose constraints based on location if organs are at risk

SYSTEMIC THERAPY

For over a decade, there were limited systemic treatment options for unresectable or advanced HCC (BCLC Stage C) with vascular invasion and/or evidence of spread outside the liver. Sorafenib, an oral multikinase inhibitor, was the first to demonstrate a survival benefit but was limited to those with good performance status and CP A cirrhosis.[41] Many agents after sorafenib's FDA approval in 2008 failed to show any survival advantages in comparison to sorafenib and therefore, sorafenib remained the first-line therapy for many years.

Fortunately, the systemic treatment landscape is rapidly evolving and advances have been made in targeted therapeutics and immunotherapies.[42] Lenvatinib, an antiangiogenic receptor tyrosine kinase inhibitor, demonstrated noninferiority against sorafenib and was approved for first-line therapy in advanced HCC in 2018.[43] Most recently, the FDA approved combination immunotherapy with atezolizumab plus bevacizumab after demonstrating superior survival compared with sorafenib and will likely become the new standard of care in unresectable HCC.[44]

Approved Second-Line Therapies
- Regorafenib- Oral tyrosine kinase inhibitor
  - First drug to show efficacy after disease progression on sorafenib
- Cabozantinib- Oral multikinase inhibitor
  - Refractory or intolerant to sorafenib
- Ramucirumab- Recombinant monoclonal antibody to vascular endothelial growth factor (VEGF) receptor 2
  - Refractory or intolerant to sorafenib with AFP >/ = 400 ng/mL
- Nivolumab- Monoclonal antibody programmed death (PD-1) inhibitor
- Pembrolizumab- Monoclonal antibody PD-1 and PD-L1 inhibitor

A variety of systemic treatment options are now available with favorable side effect profiles and will hopefully improve survival rates in patients with advanced and unresectable HCC. There are many studies underway to determine the best therapeutic options, combination therapy, and how to sequence first- and second-line therapies.

PALLIATIVE CARE

The HCC cancer continuum is a journey, which involves the patient, family, health care providers, and multiple support systems. Having knowledgeable health care providers explain options and allow time for the patient and family to make decisions decreases the burden of navigating end-of-life care choices. Palliative care and hospice are often confused, and the two types of care are often interpreted and referred to interchangeably. Hospice care is a compassionate care end of life model, which uses a team-oriented approach for medical management and coordination of emotional and spiritual care aligned with the patient's requests.[45] Hospice care is used during the last 6 months of life expectancy, offering support, dignity, comfort, and quality of life during this vulnerable time.[45] Palliative care juxtaposed to hospice care has similarities in the end-of-life care utilization; however, palliative care can be accessed earlier in the disease process and aims to promote comfort and dignity while pursuing curative treatment.[45] Nursing considerations for palliative care include mental, physical, emotional, and spiritual support. Nurses are well-positioned to meet the emotional and supportive care needs of patients with BCLC terminal Stage D HCC.

CLINICS CARE POINTS

- Early-stage HCC can be potentially cured by resection, liver transplantation, or ablation
- Resection is preferred treatment modality in single HCC (BCLC stage 0)
- Liver transplant for HCC demonstrates best overall survival in patients with portal hypertension (BCLC stage 0-A)
- Limited organ availability requires better use of nontransplant curative options for HCC
- TACE and TARE are commonly used in intermediate (BCLC stage B) HCC
- Despite advancements in systemic therapies, mortality in HCC continues to rise
- Palliative and hospice care should be considered in addition to best supportive care in BCLC D disease
- Choice of management approach in HCC is improved by multidisciplinary consensus

SUMMARY

The incidence of HCC is rapidly rising, and various treatment modalities are used to potentially cure or slow disease progression. Outcomes are dependent on tumor characteristics, general health status and hepatic function. Due to the complexity of HCC, a multidisciplinary approach including nursing is needed to successfully educate, navigate, and provide supportive care needs to patients struggling with HCC and improve their health outcomes.

DISCLOSURE

The authors have nothing to disclose.

REFERENCES

1. Marrero JA, Kulik LM, Sirlin CB, et al. Diagnosis, staging, and management of hepatocellular carcinoma: 2018 practice guidance by the American association for the study of liver diseases. Hepatology 2018;68(2):723–50.

2. Ferlay J, Colombet M, Soerjomataram I, et al. Estimating the global cancer incidence and mortality in 2018: GLOBOCAN sources and methods. Int J Cancer 2019;144(8):1941–53.
3. Heimbach JK, Kulik LM, Finn RS, et al. AASLD guidelines for the treatment of hepatocellular carcinoma. Hepatology 2018;67(1):358–80.
4. McGlynn KA, Petrick JL, El-Serag HB. Epidemiology of hepatocellular carcinoma. Hepatology 2021;73(Suppl 1):4–13.
5. Petrick JL, Florio AA, Loomba R, et al. Have incidence rates of liver cancer peaked in the United States? Cancer 2020;126(13):3151–5.
6. Duseja A. Staging of hepatocellular carcinoma. J Clin Exp Hepatol 2014;4(Suppl 3):S74–9.
7. Brar G, Greten TF, Graubard BI, et al. Hepatocellular carcinoma survival by etiology: a SEER-Medicare Database analysis. Hepatol Commun 2020;4(10): 1541–51.
8. Child CG, Turcotte JG. Surgery and portal hypertension. Major problems in clinical surgery 1964;1:1–85.
9. Durand F, Valla D. Assessment of the prognosis of cirrhosis: Child-Pugh versus MELD. J Hepatol 2005;42(Suppl 1):S100–7.
10. Durand F, Valla D. Assessment of prognosis of cirrhosis. Semin Liver Dis 2008; 28(1):110–22.
11. Kamath PS, Wiesner RH, Malinchoc M, et al. A model to predict survival in patients with end-stage liver disease. Hepatology 2001;33(2):464–70.
12. Boursier J, Cesbron E, Tropet AL, et al. Comparison and improvement of MELD and Child-Pugh score accuracies for the prediction of 6-month mortality in cirrhotic patients. J Clin Gastroenterol 2009;43(6):580–5.
13. Bialecki ES, Di Bisceglie AM. Diagnosis of hepatocellular carcinoma. HPB (Oxford) 2005;7(1):26–34.
14. Yamashita Y, Mitsuzaki K, Yi T, et al. Small hepatocellular carcinoma in patients with chronic liver damage: prospective comparison of detection with dynamic MR imaging and helical CT of the whole liver. Radiology 1996;200(1):79–84.
15. Choi JY, Lee JM, Sirlin CB. CT and MR imaging diagnosis and staging of hepatocellular carcinoma: part I. Development, growth, and spread: key pathologic and imaging aspects. Radiology 2014;272(3):635–54.
16. Choi JY, Lee JM, Sirlin CB. CT and MR imaging diagnosis and staging of hepatocellular carcinoma: part II. Extracellular agents, hepatobiliary agents, and ancillary imaging features. Radiology 2014;273(1):30–50.
17. Tang A, Bashir MR, Corwin MT, et al. Evidence supporting LI-RADS major features for CT- and MR imaging-based diagnosis of hepatocellular carcinoma: a systematic review. Radiology 2018;286(1):29–48.
18. Karademir S. "Staging of hepatocellular carcinoma.". Hepatoma Res 2018;4.
19. Edge SB, Compton CC. The American Joint Committee on Cancer: the 7th edition of the AJCC cancer staging manual and the future of TNM. Ann Surg Oncol 2010; 17(6):1471–4.
20. Llovet JM, Fuster J, Bruix J. Intention-to-treat analysis of surgical treatment for early hepatocellular carcinoma: resection versus transplantation. Hepatology 1999;30(6):1434–40.
21. Forner A, Da Fonseca LG, Díaz-González Á, et al. Controversies in the management of hepatocellular carcinoma. JHEP Rep 2019;1(1):17–29.
22. Han HS, Shehta A, Ahn S, et al. Laparoscopic versus open liver resection for hepatocellular carcinoma: Case-matched study with propensity score matching. J Hepatol 2015;63(3):643–50.

23. Tabrizian P, Jibara G, Shrager B, et al. Recurrence of hepatocellular cancer after resection: patterns, treatments, and prognosis. Ann Surg 2015;261(5):947–55.

24. Mazzaferro V, Regalia E, Doci R, et al. Liver transplantation for the treatment of small hepatocellular carcinomas in patients with cirrhosis. N Engl J Med 1996; 334(11):693–700.

25. Yao FY, Kerlan RK Jr, Hirose R, et al. Excellent outcome following down-staging of hepatocellular carcinoma prior to liver transplantation: an intention-to-treat analysis. Hepatology 2008;48(3):819–27.

26. Kulik L, Heimbach JK, Zaiem F, et al. Therapies for patients with hepatocellular carcinoma awaiting liver transplantation: a systematic review and meta-analysis. Hepatology 2018;67(1):381–400.

27. Taniguchi M, Kim SR, Imoto S, et al. Long-term outcome of percutaneous ethanol injection therapy for minimum-sized hepatocellular carcinoma. World J Gastroenterol 2008;14(13):1997–2002.

28. Shiina S, Sato K, Tateishi R, et al. Percutaneous ablation for hepatocellular carcinoma: comparison of various ablation techniques and surgery. Can J Gastroenterol Hepatol 2018;2018:4756147.

29. Germani G, Pleguezuelo M, Gurusamy K, et al. Clinical outcomes of radiofrequency ablation, percutaneous alcohol and acetic acid injection for hepatocellular carcinoma: a meta-analysis. J Hepatol 2010;52(3):380–8.

30. Abdelaziz AO, Abdelmaksoud AH, Nabeel MM, et al. Transarterial chemoembolization combined with either radiofrequency or microwave ablation in management of hepatocellular carcinoma. Asian Pac J Cancer Prev 2017;18(1):189–94.

31. Han K, Kim JH. Transarterial chemoembolization in hepatocellular carcinoma treatment: Barcelona clinic liver cancer staging system. World J Gastroenterol 2015;21(36):10327–35.

32. Young S, Craig P, Golzarian J. Current trends in the treatment of hepatocellular carcinoma with transarterial embolization: a cross-sectional survey of techniques. Eur Radiol 2019;29(6):3287–95.

33. Drott J, Björnsson B, Sandström P, et al. Experiences of symptoms and Impact on Daily life and health in hepatocellular carcinoma patients: a Meta-synthesis of Qualitative Research. Cancer Nurs 2022. https://doi.org/10.1097/NCC. 0000000000001044 [published online ahead of print, 2022 Jan 12].

34. Li H, Wu F, Duan M, et al. Drug-eluting bead transarterial chemoembolization (TACE) vs conventional TACE in treating hepatocellular carcinoma patients with multiple conventional TACE treatments history: a comparison of efficacy and safety. Medicine (Baltimore) 2019;98(21):e15314.

35. Li J, Shi C, Shi J, et al. Determination of risk factors for fever after transarterial chemoembolization with drug-eluting beads for hepatocellular carcinoma. Medicine (Baltimore) 2021;100(44):e27636.

36. Tohme S, Bou Samra P, Kaltenmeier C, et al. Radioembolization for hepatocellular carcinoma: a Nationwide 10-year experience. J Vasc Interv Radiol 2018;29(7): 912–9.e2.

37. Sacco R, Mismas V, Marceglia S, et al. Transarterial radioembolization for hepatocellular carcinoma: an update and perspectives. World J Gastroenterol 2015; 21(21):6518–25.

38. Benson AB III, Abrams TA, Ben-Josef E, et al. Hepatobiliary cancers. J Natl Compr Canc Netw 2009;7(4):350–91.

39. Huertas A, Baumann AS, Saunier-Kubs F, et al. Stereotactic body radiation therapy as an ablative treatment for inoperable hepatocellular carcinoma. Radiother Oncol 2015;115(2):211–6.

40. Bang A, Dawson LA. Radiotherapy for HCC: Ready for prime time? JHEP Rep 2019;1(2):131–7.
41. Llovet JM, Ricci S, Mazzaferro V, et al. Sorafenib in advanced hepatocellular carcinoma. N Engl J Med 2008;359(4):378–90.
42. Galle PR, Dufour JF, Peck-Radosavljevic M, et al. Systemic therapy of advanced hepatocellular carcinoma. Future Oncol 2021;17(10):1237–51.
43. von Felden J. New systemic agents for hepatocellular carcinoma: an update 2020. Curr Opin Gastroenterol 2020;36(3):177–83.
44. Kudo M. Recent advances in systemic therapy for hepatocellular carcinoma in an aging Society: 2020 update. Liver Cancer 2020;9(6):640–62.
45. Casey D. Hospice and Palliative Care: What's the Difference? MedSurg Nursing 2019;28(3):196. Available at: https://search.ebscohost.com/login.aspx?direct=true&AuthType=shib&db=edsgao&AN=edsgcl.592555588&site=eds-live&scope=site. Accessed January 28, 2022.

Variceal Bleeds in Patients with Cirrhosis

Quenell Zacharie Douglas, MSN, APRN, FNP-C

KEYWORDS

- Cirrhosis • Gastroesophageal varices • Variceal bleeding • Portal hypertension
- Endoscopy

KEY POINTS

- One of the most life-threatening complications of liver cirrhosis is acute variceal bleeding.
- Gastroesophageal varices indicate significant portal hypertension.
- Endoscopy plays a major role in acute as well as preventative management of gastroesophageal bleeding.
- Prevention of gastroesophageal bleeds involves screening, surveillance, and medication prophylaxis.

INTRODUCTION

Cirrhosis is the 11th most common cause of death and the third leading cause of death in people aged 45 to 64 years.[1] Approximately one million deaths worldwide are the result of cirrhosis. Cirrhosis occurs as a result of long-term inflammation of the liver. Chronic inflammation causes hepatic fibrosis, which leads to replacement of normal hepatic structure with hepatic nodules, resulting in liver failure. Complications of cirrhosis include development of ascites, variceal bleeding, and hepatic encephalopathy among others. These complications may occur with or without symptom development. If there are no resulting symptoms, the cirrhotic state is considered compensated and decompensated when symptoms are present. The presence of one or more complications with symptom development is an indication of progressing decompensation.[2]

The second most common complication of cirrhosis is gastroesophageal variceal (GEV) bleeding. The risk of mortality increases by 20% at 6 weeks following an acute variceal bleed.[2] Approximately one-third of cirrhosis-related deaths are attributable to GEV bleeding. Acute GEV bleeding requires multidisciplinary management involving medical, nursing, endoscopic, radiologic, and surgical interventions to prevent fatal outcomes.[1]

Gastroenterology, Southeast Louisiana Veterans Health Care System, 2400 Canal Street, New Orleans, LA 70119, USA
E-mail address: quenell.douglas@va.gov

Crit Care Nurs Clin N Am 34 (2022) 303–309
https://doi.org/10.1016/j.cnc.2022.04.006
0899-5885/22/Published by Elsevier Inc.

PATHOPHYSIOLOGY

Portal hypertension (PH) is a serious complication of cirrhosis and can cause formation of GEVs, among other complications. Varices are unusually dilated veins in the submucosa of the gastrointestinal (GI) tract and can occur in the esophagus, stomach, and rectum.[3] PH is defined as an increase in portal pressure causing obstruction or increased resistance of blood flow at any level within the portal venous system. Normal portal venous pressure ranges between 7 and 12 mm Hg. Portal vein pressure can be determined by measuring the pressure gradient between the portal vein and the inferior vena cava; this is called the hepatic venous pressure gradient (HVPG) and reflects actual liver portal perfusion pressure. A normal HVPG is considered to be between 1 and 5 mm Hg. Values greater than 5 indicate PH and values greater than 10 indicate clinically significant PH. PH is confirmed by the presence of GEVs seen on upper endoscopy or other abdominal portosystemic collaterals seen on imaging.[4,5]

PH is classified according to the location of obstruction in relation to the liver (**Table 1**). Prehepatic PH results when the obstruction occurs before reaching the liver. Intrahepatic PH results when the obstruction occurs within the liver itself. Posthepatic PH results when the obstruction occurs after the liver. Intrahepatic PH can further be broken down into subclasses according to the location of the obstruction within the hepatic sinusoid: presinusoidal, sinusoidal, or postsinusoidal.[5]

Cirrhosis is the most common cause of sinusoidal PH. In sinusoidal PH, obstruction is caused by structural changes (sinusoidal fibrosis and regenerative nodules) to hepatic sinusoids, which result in decreased production of vasodilators from sinusoidal cells, leading to vasoconstriction of intrahepatic circulation. Patients with sinusoidal PH typically present with splenomegaly, GEVs, collaterals, variceal bleeds, ascites, and hepatic encephalopathy.[5]

BACKGROUND

The development of varices is an indication of the increasing severity of cirrhosis. Varices are more often seen in patients who have Child-Turcotte-Pugh (CTP) scores of class C (85%) as compared with CTP class A (40%).[1] Esophageal varices (EV) have a greater occurrence rate than gastric varices (GV). Esophageal varices may be found in approximately 50% to 60% of patients with compensated cirrhosis and approximately 85% of patients with decompensated cirrhosis.[6] Gastric varices are seen in 15% to 20% of patients with portal hypertension. Although GV only account for 10% to 30% of variceal bleeds, they have a higher rate of rebleeding and transfusion requirements and are associated with greater mortality rates.[1]

Esophageal varices are most often observed in the lower 2 to 5 cm of the esophagus. Gastric varices are classified into 4 types according to their location and relation to esophageal varices. Sarin classification is most commonly used to classify the different types of GV (**Fig. 1**).[6] The most common type of GV is type GOV1, and it accounts for approximately 75% of GV. With this type, esophageal varices extend below the cardia into the lesser curvature of the stomach. In type GOV2, esophageal varices extend into the greater curvature of the stomach and account for approximately 21% of GV. Isolated GV type 1 are found in the fundus, whereas isolated GV type 1 may be seen anywhere in the stomach of duodenum. Isolated GV are less common and account for approximately 2% to 7% of variceal bleeds.[1]

Table 1
Portal hypertension classification

Type	Most Common Causes	Clinical Presentation	Hemodynamic Characteristics
Prehepatic	Portal vein occlusion (thrombosis or neoplasm) Splenic vein occlusion (thrombosis or neoplasm) Portal vein stenosis	Splenomegaly GEVs Collaterals Variceal bleeding	Normal HVPG Normal WHVP Normal FHVP
Intrahepatic			
Presinusoidal	Schistosomiasis Primary biliary cholangitis (early stage) Primary sclerosing cholangitis Focal nodular hyperplasia Idiopathic PH Sarcoidosis	Splenomegaly GEVs Collaterals Variceal bleeding	Normal HVPG Normal or slightly elevated WHVP Normal FHVP
Sinusoidal	Cirrhosis (viral, alcoholic, NASH-related) Alcoholic hepatitis Primary biliary cholangitis (advanced stages)	Splenomegaly GEVs Collateral Variceal bleeding Ascites Hepatic encephalopathy	Elevated HVPG Elevated WHVP Normal FHVP
Postsinusoidal	Venoocclusive disease	Splenomegaly Collateral Ascites	Normal HVPG Elevated WHVP Elevated FHVP
Posthepatic			
Vascular obstruction	Hepatic vein thrombosis (Budd-Chiari syndrome)	Ascites Intrahepatic collaterals	Not possible to catheterize hepatic veins
Liver congestion	Chronic right heart failure Chronic constrictive pericarditis Restrictive cardiomyopathy Tricuspid insufficiency	Ascites	Normal HVPG Elevated WHVP Elevated FHVP

Abbreviations: FHVP, free hepatic venous pressure; NASH, nonalcoholic steatohepatitis; WHVP, wedged hepatic venous pressure.
From Turco L, Garcia-Tsao G. Portal hypertension pathogenesis and diagnosis. Clinics in Liver Disease. 2019;23(4):577; with permission.

DISCUSSION

Variceal bleeds can cause hemodynamic instability. Therapeutic interventions for management of acute GEV bleeding are aimed at restoration of hemostasis. Initial management of acute GEV bleeding involves utilization of basic life support measures that focus on resuscitation of airway, breathing, and circulation. Patients presenting with accompanying hepatic encephalopathy are at an increased risk of aspiration of blood and gastric contents. Measures such as endotracheal intubation should be initiated to protect the airway and ensure proper breath ventilation. Intravenous access should be initiated to manage resultant hypovolemia and hypotension with infusion of crystalloid fluids and transfusion of blood products. Systolic blood pressure should

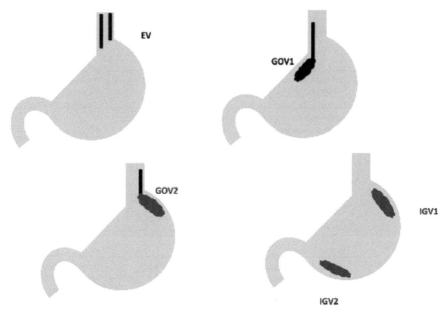

Fig. 1. Classification of gastroesophageal varices. (*From* Jakab SS, Garcia-Tsao G. Evaluation and management of esophageal and gastric varices in patients with cirrhosis. Clinics in Liver Disease. 2020;24:336; with permission.)

be maintained greater than 100 mm Hg. If hemoglobin values are less than 7 g/dL, transfusion of red blood cells is required to maintain a hemoglobin level between 7 and 9 g/dL.[1]

THERAPEUTIC OPTIONS

Pharmacologic, endoscopic, and sometimes surgical therapy are used to control acute variceal bleeding. Vasoactive medications aimed at decreasing portal pressure, such as octreotide, are used; this is given as a continuous infusion for up to 5 days. The administration of vasoactive drugs decreases the 7-day all-cause mortality. One study has shown that vasoactive drugs alone can stop bleeding by as much as 83%. Patients with an acute GI bleed are also at risk of developing bacterial infections such as peritonitis, bacteremia, urinary tract infection, and pneumonia. Infection can decrease the ability to control bleeding and increase the risk of death. Prophylactic antibiotics such as quinolones and third-generation cephalosporins are recommended to reduce the risk of infection and improve mortality. They should be administered for a total of 7 days.[3,4] Studies have shown that use of prophylactic antibiotics during an acute variceal bleed have led to a decrease in development of bacterial infections, mortality, and rebleeding rates, as well as decreased hospital admission time.[1]

Endoscopic evaluation with esophagogastroduodenoscopy (EGD) should be performed within 12 hours of admission. Studies have shown that combining pharmacotherapy along with endoscopic therapy has the potential for greater control of bleeding and lowers rebleed risk at 5 days. Endoscopic variceal ligation (EVL) is used as first-line therapy for esophageal and GOV1 varices. Multiple bands are applied to the distal 8 cm portion of the esophagus until varices are decompressed or until placement becomes too proximal. EVL is effective at controlling variceal bleeding in approximately

90% of cases. Complications associated with EVL may be seen in approximately 2% to 20% of patients. These complications include dysphagia, retrosternal pain, esophageal stricture, ulcerations, perforation, infection, and sometimes rebleeding.

In the event of uncontrolled variceal bleeding or patients who are not candidates for EVL, endoscopic injection sclerotherapy, balloon tamponade, and transjugular intrahepatic portosystemic shunt (TIPS) may be used for salvage therapy. Sclerotherapy is a technique where a sclerosant solution (liquid containing an irritant that causes inflammation and thrombosis) is injected into or very near the bleeding varix. Sclerotherapy is not without its issues. Approximately 40% of patients undergoing sclerotherapy develop complications such as esophageal ulcerations, strictures, and hemothorax, among others. Balloon tamponade uses a Sengstaken-Blakemore tube. Hemostasis is achieved in approximately 50% to 80% of cases using this method; however, it has a high rebleed rate of approximately 50% after balloons are deflated. Balloon tamponade is also associated with several complications, particularly, aspiration pneumonia. TIPS involves creation of an intrahepatic shunt placed between the portal and hepatic veins and is usually performed by an interventional radiologist. TIPS redirects blood flow, thereby decreasing portal venous pressure. Bleeding is controlled in 95% of TIPS cases. The rebleed rate is 18%. Although TIPS offers a high rate of hemostasis, it too has complications; most notably, it can cause hepatic encephalopathy.[1,3,7]

EVL and injection sclerotherapy are not recommended for treatment of IGV type varices. Glue injection with cyanoacrylate is the first-line treatment of these types of varices. Cessation of bleeding in patients is achieved in 50% to 100% of cases and prevention of rebleed in 0% to 40% of cases.[7]

CLINICAL OUTCOMES

One year after an acute variceal bleed, the rate of rebleeding is 60% and mortality rate 33%. Use of a nonselective beta blocker (NSBB), such as propranolol, along with routine EGD surveillance should be done following an acute GI bleed in patients who have not undergone TIPS. Nonselective β-blockers decrease portal pressure by inhibiting β_2-induced splanchnic vasodilation, resulting in reduced portal venous flow. The therapeutic goal for the use of NSBB is a resting heart rate of 55 to 60 bpm and a systolic blood pressure greater than 90 mm Hg. The NSBB is titrated up to achieve the therapeutic goal. The initial surveillance EGD should be scheduled 1 to 2 weeks following index treatment of acute variceal bleeds, followed by repeat EGD at 4- to 6-week intervals until obliteration of varices. For patients having undergone TIPS, an ultrasound with doppler assessment to monitor TIPS patency every 6 months along with consideration for liver transplantation is recommended.[1,3,4]

Primary prophylaxis for prevention of an initial GEV bleed is recommended for patients at increased risk of bleeding, which includes patients with medium, large, or giant GEVs; patients with small varices with red wale marks (sign of recent hemorrhage) seen on EGD; and decompensated patients with small varices. The American Associated for Study of Liver Diseases recommends an EGD to evaluate for GEVs at the time of cirrhosis diagnosis. Endoscopy helps guide decision-making for management of GEV by identifying absence of varices and if present, estimating the size of varices: small (<5 mm), medium to large (>5 mm), or giant (>10 mm). If GEV are not seen initially, surveillance EGD can be performed every 2 to 3 years. If varices less than 5 mm are found, surveillance EGD should be performed every 1 to 2 years. For small varices considered high risk (CTP class C or red wale sign), addition of NSBBs is recommended. Surveillance EGD for those with decompensated cirrhosis and varices less than 5 mm should be performed annually. Either the use of NSBB or EVL can be used for management of medium and large-sized GEVs. Studies evaluating the use of NSBB or EVL alone compared with combination therapy with both have shown combination use is more effective than single use.[1,3]

EGD is the gold standard for GEV screening; however, noninvasive tests have been used to predict the presence of GEV with subpar results. Noninvasive testing also does not correlate well with HPVG changes. The more recent development of a noninvasive test known as transient elastography (TE) measurement allows for early detection of patients with chronic liver disease at risk for development of clinically significant portal hypertension. There is an excellent correlation between the HVPG and liver stiffness score in patients with advanced liver fibrosis and cirrhosis. Liver stiffness score (LS) of greater than 13.6 kPa or LS greater than 21 kPa have been found to have 90% sensitivity and a 90% specificity for the diagnosis of clinically significant portal hypertension. The combination of TE measurement (LS < 20 kPa) and platelet count (>150,000/mm^3) has recently been recommended to identify compensated cirrhotic patients with a very low probability (<5%) of developing high-risk GEVs, potentially preventing the need to undergo endoscopy.[3,8]

SUMMARY

Cirrhosis is the 11th most common cause of death and the third leading cause of death in people aged 45 to 64 years. PH is a serious complication of cirrhosis and can cause GEVs, among other complications. GEV bleeding is one of the most fatal complications of cirrhosis, causing increased morbidity and mortality rates. The single most important measure to prevent GEV bleeding is to start primary prophylaxis measures aimed at prevention of the initial GEV bleed, which involves utilization of screening, surveillance, and pharmacologic measures.

When an acute GEV bleed does occur, it is imperative to intervene promptly to help prevent fatal outcomes. After 1 year of an acute variceal bleed, the rate of rebleeding is 60% and mortality rate 33%. Once an acute GEV has occurred, secondary prevention measures to prevent rebleeding must be initiated. These measures include use of an NSBB along with routine EGD surveillance.[1–3]

CLINICS CARE POINTS

- On initial diagnosis of cirrhosis, patients should be evaluated to determine the stage or degree of hepatic fibrosis along with state of compensation and assess for the presence of portal hypertension and resultant complications such as GEVs.
- Patients at high risk for development of GEVs should begin primary prophylaxis to prevent an initial GEV bleed: EGD to evaluate for GEVs and initiation of NSBBs.
- In the event of an acute GEV bleed, immediate measures to control bleeding include restoration of hemostasis, pharmacologic treatment with vasoactive medications to decrease portal pressure, endoscopic management with EVL, and sometimes surgical therapy.
- Following an acute GEV, secondary measures must be initiated to prevent rebleeding: use of an NSBB along with routine EGD surveillance.

DEDICATION

This article is dedicated to Derrel J. Zacharie.

ACKNOWLEDGMENTS

I would like to acknowledge Cynthia Benz DNP APRN for her assistance with the research for this article and encouragement to complete this opportunity.

DISCLOSURE

The author has nothing to disclose.

REFERENCES

1. Tayyem O, Balil M, Samuel R, et al. Evaluation and management of variceal bleeding. Dis – a – Month 2018;64:312–20.
2. Gines P, Krag A, Abraldes J, et al. Lancet 2021;98:1359–76.
3. Kovacs TO, Jensen DM. Varices, esophageal, gastric and rectal. Clin Liver Dis 2019;23:625–42.
4. Simonetto DA, Liu M, Kamath PS. Portal hypertension and related complications: diagnosis and management. Mayo Clin Proc 2019;94(4):714–26.
5. Turco L, Garcia-Tsao G. Portal hypertension pathogenesis and diagnosis. Clin Liver Dis 2019;23:573–87.
6. Jakab SS, Garcia-Tsao G. Evaluation and management of esophageal and gastric varices in patients with cirrhosis. Clin Liver Dis 2020;24:335–50.
7. Nett A, Binmoeller KF. Endoscopic management of portal hypertension – related bleeding. Gastrointest Endosc Clin N America 2019;29:321–37.
8. Mauro E, Gadano A. What's new in portal hypertension? Liver Int 2020;40(Suppi.1): 122–7.

Management of the Adult Patient with Cirrhosis Complicated by Ascites

Anna M. Nobbe, MSN[a],*, Heather M. McCurdy, MSN[b]

KEYWORDS

- Cirrhosis • Ascites • Sodium restriction • Paracentesis • TIPS

KEY POINTS

- Ascites is often the first and is the most common complication of cirrhosis, with an accompanying significant reduction in life expectancy.
- New-onset ascites requires a diagnostic paracentesis, including calculation of a serum ascites albumin gradient (SAAG); a SAAG greater than 1.1 g/dL is highly suggestive of portal hypertension.
- Sodium restriction and diuretics are the mainstay of management; however, recurrent or refractory ascites may require large volume paracentesis or creation of a transjugular intrahepatic portosystemic shunt.
- Secondary complications of ascites include refractory ascites, hyponatremia, and hepatorenal syndrome and are associated with reduced survival.
- Patients with ascites should be considered for liver transplant (LT), and if not candidates are referred for palliative care.

INTRODUCTION

The most common complication of cirrhosis is ascites, and this leads to a reduction in overall survival and quality of life. Providers caring for patients with cirrhosis must be attuned to patient complaints such as peripheral edema, abdominal distension, and weight gain in order to diagnose the condition right away and initiate treatment, if indicated. Mild-to-moderate ascites is managed with dietary sodium restriction and judicious use of diuretics. Tense ascites often requires a large volume paracentesis (LVP) accompanied by an albumin infusion, in addition to sodium restriction and diuretics as tolerated. Recurrent and/or refractory ascites may require serial paracenteses or

[a] Department of Digestive Diseases, Cincinnati VA Medical Center, 3200 Vine Street (111-GI), Cincinnati, OH 45220, USA; [b] Gastroenterology Section, VA Ann Arbor Healthcare System, 2215 Fuller Road (111D), Ann Arbor, MI 48105, USA
* Corresponding author.
E-mail address: Anna.Nobbe@va.gov
Twitter: @amarieNP (A.M.N.); @hmccurdyNP (H.M.M.)

Crit Care Nurs Clin N Am 34 (2022) 311–320
https://doi.org/10.1016/j.cnc.2022.04.005
0899-5885/22/Published by Elsevier Inc.

ccnursing.theclinics.com

creation of a transjugular intrahepatic portosystemic shunt (TIPS). Because of the possible additional complications seen with ascites, inpatient providers must also evaluate the hospitalized patient with cirrhosis and ascites for infection of ascitic fluid, for metabolic derangements related to diuretic use, and for acute kidney injury (AKI), regardless of reason for admission. Finally, patients with ascites should be considered for liver transplant, and if not, candidates for transplant should be referred for palliative care.

Natural History and Prognosis

Ascites develops in greater than 50% of patients with cirrhosis within 10 years of diagnosis.[1] Portal pressure in the early stage of cirrhosis may be normal; however, it increases as the underlying disease progresses, leading to clinically significant portal hypertension.[2] An increase in portal pressure and decrease in liver function may lead to ascites formation, portal hypertensive gastrointestinal bleeding, hepatic encephalopathy (HE), and jaundice. The development of any of these complications signifies the transition from "compensated" to "decompensated" cirrhosis (**Fig. 1**). Ascites is often the first and is the most common complication of cirrhosis, occurring in 5% to 10% of patients per year, with an accompanying significant reduction in life expectancy—from an 80% 5-year survival rate to only 30%.[3] Median survival in patients with compensated cirrhosis is > 12 years, whereas that of patients with decompensated cirrhosis is approximately 2 years.[4] The reduction in survival seems to be related to the development of additional complications, such as refractory ascites, hyponatremia, and hepatorenal syndrome (HRS), which are each associated with reduced survival.[5] If appropriate, patients with ascites should be referred for liver transplant evaluation, given that the long-term prognosis is poor. However, patients may remain on the liver transplant waitlist for a long period of time without ever being offered a donor organ.[5] Patients with alcohol-induced cirrhosis who achieve sustained alcohol abstinence may have improvement in liver function and resolution of ascites; this may be true as well with eradication of hepatitis C or viral suppression of hepatitis B.[2]

Definitions

Uncomplicated ascites is neither infected nor associated with HRS.[1] In its mildest form—detectable only by ultrasound—ascites is termed *Grade 1*. Moderate, or *Grade 2*, ascites is discernible by visible distension of the abdomen. Marked, or tense, abdominal distension signifies *Grade 3* ascites.

Recurrent ascites is ascites that recurs on at least 3 occasions within a 12-month period despite dietary sodium restriction and adequate diuretics or requires 3 or greater LVP within 1 year.[2,3]

Refractory ascites is defined by the International Ascites Club as ascites that "cannot be mobilized or the early occurrence of which cannot be satisfactorily prevented by medical therapy".[6]

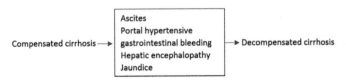

Compensated cirrhosis ⟶ | Ascites
Portal hypertensive
gastrointestinal bleeding
Hepatic encephalopathy
Jaundice | ⟶ Decompensated cirrhosis

Fig. 1. "Compensated" to "decompensated" cirrhosis.

DISCUSSION
Diagnosis

It is important to take a thorough medical history when assessing the patient with ascites. This should include patient's risk factors for chronic liver disease (viral hepatitis, alcohol use, metabolic factors, and family history of liver disease) and reported symptoms and impact on quality of life. Earlier studies have demonstrated that a patient's history and symptoms can often accurately predict both the presence and the absence of ascites. There are key elements on which to focus: a perceived increase in abdominal girth, weight gain, clothing feeling tight in the waist, peripheral edema, early satiety, shortness of breath, and nonspecific abdominal discomfort.[7] Onset of the above symptoms is also important and helps differentiate between ascites and obesity, for example, rapid weight gain is more likely to be ascites. Ascites typically develops over weeks, different from obesity, which develops during months or even years.[8]

The findings on physical examination can also assist in the diagnosis of ascites but is relatively insensitive if fewer than 1,500 mL of ascitic fluid present. Key elements of the physical examination include bulging flanks, shifting dullness, a fluid wave, and peripheral edema.[7,8] In the case of a patient with new-onset ascites, who is not already known to have cirrhosis, the provider must also assess for other physical stigmata of cirrhosis (splenomegaly, muscle wasting, clubbing, palmar erythema, gynecomastia, abdominal wall collaterals, or spider angioma) because this will narrow the differential diagnosis of ascites.[3]

The initial evaluation of a patient with new-onset ascites should include abdominal ultrasound. Patients with known cirrhosis who are undergoing serial ultrasounds for hepatocellular carcinoma surveillance may have an incidental finding of ascites on their imaging studies. Newly discovered ascites requires paracentesis (if there is enough accessible fluid to sample) and ascitic fluid analysis to determine if cirrhosis is the cause.

A paracentesis is a procedure that involves removing ascitic fluid from the peritoneal cavity using a sterile technique.[9] There are essentially 2 types of paracenteses: diagnostic and therapeutic. No matter how obvious the cause is, a diagnostic paracentesis should be performed in patients with new-onset grade 2 or grade 3 ascites. A diagnostic paracentesis should also be performed in patients with cirrhosis and ascites on admission to the hospital, even if patients do not display symptoms.[3,8] An initial diagnostic paracentesis involves the removal of a small amount of ascitic fluid that is sent for a battery of tests, such as ascitic fluid neutrophil count, ascitic fluid total protein, and ascitic fluid albumin. A serum albumin is also obtained in order to calculate the serum ascites albumin gradient (SAAG). SAAG 1.1 g/dL or greater is highly suggestive of portal hypertension as the cause of ascites. Other tests may be necessary depending on the patient's clinical history, such as glucose concentration, lactate dehydrogenase, cytology, and amylase concentration. These tests assist in determining the cause of the ascites. SAAG 1.1 g/dL or lesser essentially excludes portal hypertension as the cause; potential causes may instead be peritoneal carcinomatosis or other clinical conditions. Once cirrhosis has been determined to be the cause for ascites, future diagnostic paracentesis to rule out spontaneous bacterial peritonitis (SBP) may only require ascitic fluid neutrophil count.[3]

Treatment/Management

Sodium restriction

Grade 1 ascites generally requires no treatment other than the reduction of sodium intake. Because renal sodium retention is the driving force behind ascites formation, inducing a negative sodium balance is the primary goal of treatment.[5] Restricting sodium intake to no more than 2g daily allows for adequate renal sodium excretion, whereas the addition of diuretics leads to an increase in renal sodium output.[3] Dietary salt restriction alone leads to the resolution of ascites in 10% to 15% of patients.[10] Although patients often prefer LVP for immediate relief of moderate or grade 2 ascites, sodium restriction combined with diuretics is the preferred initial way to manage ascites in the outpatient setting.

A sodium-restricted diet can be challenging because patients are often told to reduce dietary sodium by "throwing away the salt shaker" and "avoiding processed foods." This advice is simplistic and may not be useful if there is poor access to quality food sources or food insecurity. Concrete written examples of what foods to avoid and how to make food substitutions are recommended and referral for nutrition counseling should be considered.

A diet that is lower in sodium may be unpalatable, leading to reduced oral intake, at a time when patients with cirrhosis should maximize nutrition to avoid malnutrition, frailty, and sarcopenia.[11] Abdominal distension may lead to early satiety and anorexia as well. Patients should avoid salt substitutes because they often contain potassium, which may lead to hyperkalemia due to concomitant potassium-sparing diuretic use.[5]

Diuretics

Diuretics increase renal sodium excretion, and this leads to passive water excretion.[5] The aldosterone antagonist spironolactone is used primarily, with or without the addition of the loop diuretic furosemide. In practice, the medications often are initiated at the same time, for simplification of administration and patient education. The initial starting dosages are spironolactone 50-100 mg/d + furosemide 20-40 mg/d, taken together, and can be titrated upward to a maximum of spironolactone 400 mg/d + furosemide 160 mg/d. Patients should be monitored for the development of adverse effects (eg, dehydration, confusion, or even gynecomastia, which is specific to spironolactone), or changes in serum sodium, potassium, and/or AKI. AKI, or the increase of creatinine by at least 0.3 mg/dL in 48 hours is related to loop diuretic usage. Hyponatremia and hypokalemia may also occur with loop diuretics. Hyperkalemia, however, may occur with an aldosterone antagonist that is unopposed by a loop diuretic. Many patients with adverse effects require dose reduction or discontinuation of diuretics.[12]

Patients are advised to weigh themselves daily, with a net loss goal of less than 1 kg/d if peripheral edema is present but no more than 0.5 kg/d if no peripheral edema is present.[1] Approximately, 400 mL/d ascites can be resorbed from the abdomen; therefore, adjustments to diuretics can be made every few days.[5] It is important to ascertain whether a patient is also adequately restricting sodium. Dietary recall can be unreliable, and patients may not report (or understand) their dietary intake. A spot urine sample to check a (Na)/K ratio is very useful to determine whether a patient should respond to diuretics; a ratio greater than 1 predicts adequate renal sodium excretion in 90% of patients. Adequate sodium excretion without weight loss reflects noncompliance with sodium restriction.[13]

Large volume paracentesis

A therapeutic LVP typically is used as the initial treatment when a patient presents with symptomatic large volume or tense ascites to rapidly resolve the large volume. Serial LVP is the first-line treatment of refractory ascites.[1,8] This is a safe and effective treatment when accompanied by an albumin infusion to prevent complications associated with postparacentesis circulatory dysfunction (PPCD) such as renal impairment and hyponatremia. There is no predetermined limit to the amount of ascitic fluid that can be removed during a single procedure; however, the risk of PPCD increases when more than 8L is removed. The American Association for the Study of Liver Diseases (AASLD) practice guidance document recommends an albumin infusion of 6 to 8 g/ L of fluid, when fluid removal is more than 5L. This will help to mitigate the risk of PPCD.[14] Although LVP is a treatment option for recurrent or refractory ascites, it plays no role in the pathophysiological mechanism by which ascites develops, and therefore, the ascitic fluid will reaccumulate. Serial LVPs generally are required for patient comfort and may vary in frequency and volume.[8]

Transjugular intrahepatic portosystemic shunt

A TIPS is an intervention that can be used to treat recurrent or refractory ascites and, more specifically, treats the underlying portal hypertension. A TIPS procedure involves the placement of a stent by an interventional radiologist. The stent creates a shunt between the portal vein and hepatic vein. This aids in decompressing the liver by connecting a high-pressure system (the portal vein) to a lower pressure system (hepatic vein). The blood essentially bypasses the liver. Bypassing the liver can lead to complications such as HE or a decline in overall liver function due to a decrease in liver perfusion.[15]

TIPS is an effective treatment of recurrent or refractory ascites when patients are carefully selected. An evaluation to assess if the patient is an appropriate candidate for elective, TIPS should be completed when a patient requires frequent LVP for tense ascites (at least 3 LVP in 12 months).[1,2] Because TIPS placement reduces the portal pressure, it has a direct impact on the pathophysiological mechanism that leads to the development of ascites. Therefore, it is a more effective treatment than serial LVP.[8] It is important to discuss with the patient that the resolution of ascites after TIPS is not immediate and can take 4 to 6 months; therefore, the patient should continue to adhere to a low-sodium diet and may still require diuretics, with close monitoring.[16] Eighty percent of patients will have resolution of ascites after TIPS.[17]

A randomized study found patients who underwent a TIPS had an improved 1-year survival rate (without transplant) of 93% compared with 52% who had serial LVP. Although TIPS patients are at a higher risk of HE, there was no significant difference in the incidence between the 2 groups.[18] It is becoming apparent that patients with ascites should be evaluated for TIPS much earlier in their clinical course.

One of the primary keys to a successful elective TIPS is patient selection. The Advance Liver Therapeutic Approaches Consortium recently developed recommendations to guide the clinical practice of TIPS. This included multiple absolute contraindications to elective TIPS creation (**Box 1**).[19] There are many factors to consider during the candidacy evaluation, including the patients' model for end-stage liver disease (MELD) score, which is the strongest predictor of 90-day mortality after TIPS. Patients with a MELD score of greater than 15 have a higher rate of death, whereas patients with a MELD score of greater than 18 are considered poor candidates.[20,21] Ultimately, there is no specific MELD cut-off value, and the decision should be made by a multidisciplinary team.[19] Other factors such as a history of HE, advanced age, cardiopulmonary insufficiency, and sarcopenia should also be considered.[3,22] If a patient is determined to be a poor candidate for TIPS due to significant liver dysfunction, liver transplant should be considered.[3]

COMPLICATIONS
Refractory Ascites

Approximately 5% to 10% of patients with cirrhosis and ascites develop refractory ascites that recurs despite dietary sodium restriction and maximal diuretic therapy and

---

Box 1
Absolute contraindications to elective transjugular intrahepatic portosystemic shunt (TIPS)

- Severe congestive heart failure
- Severe untreated valvular heart disease
- Moderate-sever pulmonary hypertension despite medical optimization
- Uncontrolled systemic infection
- Refractory overt hepatic encephalopathy
- Unrelieved biliary obstruction
- Lesions or tumors in the liver parenchyma that precludes TIPS creation
- *There is no set absolute model for end-stage liver disease cutoff value*

From Boike JR, Thornburg BG, Asrani SK, et al. North American Practice-Based Recommendations for Transjugular Intrahepatic Portosystemic Shunts in Portal Hypertension [published online ahead of print, 2021 Jul 15]. Clin Gastroenterol Hepatol. 2021;S1542-3565(21)00749-7.

---

requires serial LVP.[1] This development portends poor survival, that is, 50% at 6 months.[3] Adverse effects (eg, AKI, HE, hyponatremia and/or hyperkalemia, muscle cramps) may limit the ability of the provider to use maximum dosages of diuretics.

Dietary sodium restriction remains a cornerstone of management for all stages of ascites and will help reduce the rate of ascites accumulation. Treatment of refractory or recurrent ascites is serial LVP, along with albumin infusion, with the addition of diuretics as tolerated. Fluid restriction in an attempt to manage fluid overload is not indicated unless hyponatremia is present. Selected patients with recurrent or refractory ascites may be candidates for TIPS if the frequency of LVP is required more than 3 times per year.[2]

Spontaneous Bacterial Peritonitis

SBP is an infection of the ascitic fluid. It is referred to as spontaneous because it occurs in the absence of an obvious source of infection. SBP should be suspected in patients with cirrhosis who present with abdominal pain or tenderness, diarrhea, ileus, fever, hypothermia, leukocytosis, HE, AKI, and/or jaundice. Patients with esophageal variceal hemorrhage or a history of an SBP are at an increased risk for SBP.[8,23] It is important to note that as many as a third of patients with SBP are asymptomatic.[3] A diagnostic paracentesis should be performed on patients with ascites who are emergently admitted to the hospital regardless of the indication for the admission and in the absence of symptoms.[24] A diagnostic paracentesis should also be performed in the outpatient setting if a patient with ascites develops signs, symptoms, or laboratory abnormalities consistent with an infection.[3]

The diagnosis of SBP is made when the ascitic fluid polymorphonuclear (PMN) cell count is greater than 250/mm³.[3] In addition to the cell count, it is also important to obtain cultures of the ascitic fluid. The cultures should be obtained before the patient receiving the first dose of antibiotics but empirical antibiotic treatment of a patient with a PMN greater than 250/mm³ should not be delayed allowing for the culture results. A delay in diagnosis and/or treatment can lead to increased mortality.[3,25]

The first-line empirical IV antibiotic treatment of community-acquired SBP is a third-generation cephalosporin such as ceftriaxone or cefotaxime. Most commonly, 2g cefotaxime IV, every 12 hours, for 5 to 7 days.[8] The initial antibiotic treatment should be broader spectrum if there is a high likelihood of a multidrug resistant organism infection, in which case, third-generation cephalosporins are an ineffective treatment.[3,26] It is possible to evaluate the response of empirical treatment by performing a diagnostic paracentesis 48 hours after antibiotic initiation. A decrease in PMN of less than 25% from baseline is considered a lack of response. Repeat paracentesis may not be needed if the organism isolated is susceptible and the patient is clinically improving. In the setting of a lack of response, a broader spectrum treatment should be used, and abdominal imaging performed to evaluate for secondary peritonitis.[3,27] In addition to antibiotics, albumin should also be included in the treatment regimen of a patient with SBP. It plays a vital role in the prevention of AKI. The AASLD guidance recommends 1.5 g/kg on day 1 and 1 g/kg on day 3.[3]

The median survival of a patient with SBP is 9 months; 10% to 33% of patients with SBP will die during the hospitalization. There is also a 1-year probability of SBP recurrence in 69% of patients.[8,28] Due to this high probability of recurrence, there are AASLD recommendations to guide both primary and secondary prophylaxis.[3]

Hyponatremia

Hyponatremia is defined as serum Na level of 135 mEq/L or lesser and is present in 49% of patients with cirrhotic ascites.[3] Symptoms of hyponatremia are not often seen in patients with cirrhosis but may include nausea, muscle cramping, headache, lethargy, and dizziness. Mild hyponatremia (126–135 mEq/L) is often asymptomatic and requires no intervention, apart from reinforcing dietary sodium restriction, a fluid restriction and monitoring. The development of moderate (120–125 mEq/L) or severe (<120 mEq/L) hyponatremia reflects worsening cirrhosis, and patients with serum Na less than 130 mEq/L have increased risks for developing HE, HRS, and SBP.[3] The importance of this ominous laboratory finding is highlighted by its inclusion in the MELD scoring system for liver transplant allocation in 2016.[29] Treatment of hyponatremia may include fluid restriction (no more than 1000 mL/d) and reducing or stopping diuretics and laxatives. Hospitalized patients and/or patients with severe hyponatremia may receive a more severe fluid restriction and resuscitation with IV albumin.[3]

Acute Kidney Injury and Hepatorenal Syndrome

As previously stated, AKI may occur with diuretic use. It is a common finding in patients with cirrhosis and ascites and is associated with a poor prognosis; the 30-day mortality ranges from 29% to 44%.[3] Causes of AKI may include hypovolemia (from aggressive diuresis), drug-induced nephrotoxicity (eg, nonsteroidal anti-inflammatory drugs, aminoglycosides, or iodinated contrast media), or urinary tract obstruction. AKI must be treated as soon as it is recognized, first by holding diuretics and correcting hypovolemia.[3]

HRS is a severe form of AKI. It is a late complication of cirrhosis, a secondary complication occurring after ascites has developed. Reduced renal perfusion secondary to renal vasoconstriction leads to renal failure. This complication often leads to hospitalizations and is associated with high inpatient mortality (~46%) and longer lengths of stay.[3] Management includes vasoconstrictor drugs in combination with albumin, with close monitoring for side effects. Further decline in renal function may require renal replacement therapy. Patients with acute, severe HRS should be referred for urgent liver transplant evaluation.[3]

Hepatic Hydrothorax

Hepatic hydrothorax (HH) is a pleural effusion that develops in patients with cirrhosis due to a defect in the diaphragm that allows ascitic fluid to pass into the pleural space.[8] Typically, HH develops in patients with ascites but it may develop in patients without detectable ascites (9%). HH is typically unilateral, with approximately 73% to 85% occurring on the right side. Patients can have a left-sided pleural effusion (13%–17%) or less commonly, the effusion will occur bilaterally (2%–10%).[30,31] Relatively small amounts of fluid lead to patient discomfort; 1 to 2L of fluid within the pleural space will cause shortness of breath and hypoxemia.[8] Patients with HH have a poor prognosis and a 90-day posthospitalization mortality of 74%. Diagnostically, a serum to pleural fluid albumin gradient of greater than 1.1 g/dL is suggestive of HH.[31] First-line treatment for HH is similar to treatment of ascites. It consists of a sodium-restricted diet and diuretics, often in addition to serial thoracentesis due to rapid reaccumulation of fluid.[3,32] Optimal treatment of refractory or recurrent HH is TIPS creation or liver transplant. Chest tube placement is associated with an increase in mortality and should be avoided.[3]

SUMMARY

Ascites is the most common, and often first decompensating event that occurs in patients with cirrhosis. Ascites has both a high symptom burden and high mortality rate secondary to further complications. Symptoms of ascites such as increased abdominal girth, generalized abdominal pain, early satiety, and shortness of breath have a negative impact on quality of life. Treatments used to manage ascites: dietary sodium restriction, diuretics, and LVP can also have a negative impact on quality of life. Patients are faced with diet restrictions, frequent urination, close laboratory monitoring, and serial procedures, with only temporary relief provided because ultimately the portal hypertension remains. Secondary complications of ascites include refractory ascites, hyponatremia, and HRS and are associated with reduced survival. Caring for patients with ascites and the associated complications requires a multidisciplinary approach. Consideration should be given to the appropriateness and timing of referrals for elective TIPS, liver transplant, and/or palliative care.

CLINICS CARE POINTS

1. Ascites is the most common decompensating event of cirrhosis, with the highest mortality

2. Diagnostic paracentesis should be performed on all patients with new-onset ascites

3. Diagnostic paracentesis should be performed on admission to the hospital, even in the absence of symptoms suggestive of infection

4. Dietary sodium restriction and diuretics are the mainstay of treatment

5. Spot urine Na/K ratio provides information about adherence to sodium restriction

6. Serial large volume paracentesis may be required in recurrent or refractory ascites because fluid will continue to accumulate

7. Consider transjugular intrahepatic portosystemic shunt in recurrent or refractory ascites

8. Patients with ascites should be considered for liver transplantation

DISCLOSURE

The authors have nothing to disclose.

REFERENCES

1. Moore KP, Wong F, Gines P, et al. The management of ascites in cirrhosis: report on the consensus conference of the International Ascites Club. Hepatology 2003; 38(1):258–66.
2. de Franchis R, Bosch J, Garcia-Tsao G, et al. On behalf of the baveno VII faculty, BAVENO VII - renewing consensus IN portal hypertension. J Hepatol 2022;76(4): 959–74.
3. Biggins SW, Angeli P, Garcia-Tsao G, et al. Diagnosis, evaluation, and management of ascites, spontaneous bacterial peritonitis and hepatorenal syndrome: 2021 practice guidance by the american association for the study of liver diseases. Hepatology 2021;74(2):1014–48.
4. D'Amico G, Garcia-Tsao G, Pagliaro L. Natural history and prognostic indicators of survival in cirrhosis: a systematic review of 118 studies. J Hepatol 2006;44(1): 217–31.
5. Wong F. Management of ascites in cirrhosis. J Gastroenterol Hepatol 2012;27(1): 11–20.
6. Arroyo V, Ginès P, Gerbes AL, et al. Definition and diagnostic criteria of refractory ascites and hepatorenal syndrome in cirrhosis. International Ascites Club. Hepatology 1996;23(1):164–76.
7. Simel DL, Halvorsen RA Jr, Feussner JR. Quantitating bedside diagnosis: clinical evaluation of ascites. J Gen Intern Med 1988;3(5):423–8.
8. Garcia-Tsao G. Chapter 9: ascites. In: Dooley JS, Lok ASF, Garcia-Tsao G, et al, editors. Sherlock's diseases of the liver and biliary system. 13th edition. Hoboken: Wiley-Blackwell; 2018. p. 127–50.
9. Grabau CM, Crago SF, Hoff LK, et al. Performance standards for therapeutic abdominal paracentesis. Hepatology 2004;40(2):484–8.
10. Reynolds TB. Ascites. Clin Liver Dis 2000;4(1):151–vii.
11. Lai JC, Tandon P, Bernal W, et al. Malnutrition, frailty, and sarcopenia in patients with cirrhosis: 2021 practice guidance by the American association for the study of liver diseases [published correction appears in hepatology. 2021 dec;74(6):3563. Hepatology 2021;74(3):1611–44.
12. Aithal GP, Palaniyappan N, China L, et al. Guidelines on the management of ascites in cirrhosis. Gut 2021;70(1):9–29.
13. Pinto-Marques P, Vieira A. Urinary sodium/potassium ratio on random sample as a useful tool to assess diuretic-induced natriuresis on chronic liver disease-associated ascites. Am J Gastroenterol 2007;102(1):212–3.
14. Ruiz-del-Arbol L, Monescillo A, Jimenéz W, et al. Paracentesis-induced circulatory dysfunction: mechanism and effect on hepatic hemodynamics in cirrhosis. Gastroenterology 1997;113(2):579–86.
15. Bosch J, Berzigotti A. Chapter 11: portal hypertension in cirrhosis. In: Dooley JS, Lok ASF, Garcia-Tsao G, et al, editors. Sherlock's diseases of the liver and biliary system. 13th edition. Hoboken: Wiley-Blackwell; 2018. p. 180–208.
16. Rössle M. TIPS: 25 years later. J Hepatol 2013;59(5):1081–93.
17. Tan HK, James PD, Sniderman KW, et al. Long-term clinical outcome of patients with cirrhosis and refractory ascites treated with transjugular intrahepatic portosystemic shunt insertion. J Gastroenterol Hepatol 2015;30(2):389–95.
18. Bureau C, Thabut D, Oberti F, et al. Transjugular intrahepatic portosystemic shunts with covered stents increase transplant-free survival of patients with cirrhosis and recurrent ascites [published correction appears in gastroenterology. Gastroenterology 2017;152(1):157–63.

19. Boike JR, Thornburg BG, Asrani SK, et al. North American practice-based recommendations for transjugular intrahepatic portosystemic shunts in portal hypertension [published online ahead of print, 2021 Jul 15]. Clin Gastroenterol Hepatol 2021. S1542-3565(21)00749-757.

20. Salerno F, Cammà C, Enea M, et al. Transjugular intrahepatic portosystemic shunt for refractory ascites: a meta-analysis of individual patient data [published correction appears in Gastroenterology. Gastroenterology 2007;133(3):825–34.

21. Bhogal HK, Sanyal AJ. Using transjugular intrahepatic portosystemic shunts for complications of cirrhosis. Clin Gastroenterol Hepatol 2011;9(11):936-e123.

22. Schindler P, Heinzow H, Trebicka J, et al. Shunt-induced hepatic encephalopathy in TIPS: current Approaches and clinical challenges. J Clin Med 2020;9(11):3784.

23. Bajaj JS, Kamath PS, Reddy KR. The evolving challenge of infections in cirrhosis. N Engl J Med 2021;384(24):2317–30.

24. European Association for the Study of the Liver. EASL clinical practice guidelines on the management of ascites, spontaneous bacterial peritonitis, and hepatorenal syndrome in cirrhosis. J Hepatol 2010;53(3):397–417.

25. Kim JJ, Tsukamoto MM, Mathur AK, et al. Delayed paracentesis is associated with increased in-hospital mortality in patients with spontaneous bacterial peritonitis. Am J Gastroenterol 2014;109(9):1436–42.

26. Fernández J, Acevedo J, Castro M, et al. Prevalence and risk factors of infections by multiresistant bacteria in cirrhosis: a prospective study. Hepatology 2012; 55(5):1551–61.

27. Fernández J, Bert F, Nicolas-Chanoine MH. The challenges of multi-drug-resistance in hepatology. J Hepatol 2016;65(5):1043–54.

28. Tító L, Rimola A, Ginès P, et al. Recurrence of spontaneous bacterial peritonitis in cirrhosis: frequency and predictive factors. Hepatology 1988;8(1):27–31.

29. Biggins SW. Use of serum sodium for liver transplant graft allocation: a decade in the making, now is it ready for primetime? Liver Transpl 2015;21(3):279–81.

30. Strauss RM, Boyer TD. Hepatic hydrothorax. Semin Liver Dis 1997;17(3):227–32.

31. Badillo R, Rockey DC. Hepatic hydrothorax: clinical features, management, and outcomes in 77 patients and review of the literature. Medicine (Baltimore) 2014; 93(3):135–42.

32. Garioud A, Cadranel JF, Pauwels A, et al. Albumin use in patients with cirrhosis in France: results of the "ALBU-LIVE" survey: a case for better EASL guidelines diffusion and/or revision. J Clin Gastroenterol 2017;51(9):831–8.

Hepatorenal Syndrome
From the Beginning to Now

Latanja L. Divens, PhD, DNP, APRN, FNP-BC,
Sherry L. Rivera, DNP, APRN, ANP-C, FNKF*

KEYWORDS

- Hepatorenal syndrome • Cirrhosis • Acute kidney injury

KEY POINTS

- This article discusses the hallmarks and pathophysiology of hepatorenal syndrome (HRS) and the new guidelines for the diagnosis of the condition.
- The article also highlights the significant complications and rationales for the ensuing negative effects of HRS.
- The article presents advances in the treatment of HRS from the time that the disease was first identified, including evidence-based modalities and treatments on the horizon.

HEPATORENAL SYNDROME: FROM THE BEGINNING TO NOW

End-stage liver disease is a complex disorder that is common in individuals with various conditions both acute and chronic that result in Cirrhosis. One of the most serious and devastating resulting conditions of Cirrhosis is hepatorenal syndrome (HRS). New developments regarding HRS which are now referred to as HRS-acute kidney injury (HRS-AKI) or HRS-acute kidney disease (HRS-AKD). The condition is a complex syndrome that is a direct result of vasoconstriction secondary to the gross, irreversible scarring of the liver, which leads to both structural and functional abnormalities of the liver. The disease is complex and without prompt treatment the prognosis is poor. The purpose of this article is to discuss the hallmarks and pathophysiology of HRS, the new guidelines for the diagnosis of the condition, to highlight the significant complications and rationales for the ensuing negative effects of HRS, and to present advances in the treatment of HRS from the time that the disease was first identified, including evidence-based modalities and treatments on the horizon.

Louisiana State University Health New Orleans, School of Nursing, 1900 Gravier Street, New Orleans, LA 70112, USA
* Corresponding author.
E-mail address: srive4@lsuhsc.edu

Crit Care Nurs Clin N Am 34 (2022) 321–329
https://doi.org/10.1016/j.cnc.2022.04.010
0899-5885/22/© 2022 Elsevier Inc. All rights reserved.

BACKGROUND

Hepatorenal Syndrome (HRS) is defined as a multifactorial and significantly complex syndrome that affects both the liver and kidneys. HRS results from severe scarring of the liver and additional disorders associated with Cirrhosis including Portal Hypertension (PHTN), systemic inflammation, vasodilation, and vasoconstriction that disrupt both the structure and function of the liver. AKI is a severe complication of Cirrhosis that occurs in approximately 50% of hospitalized individuals.[1] The sequence of events triggered by Cirrhosis often results in kidney dysfunction. The classic signs of HRS are prerenal azotemia, reversible vasoconstriction, and peripheral arterial vasodilation.[2] There are 2 types of the syndrome HRS-CKD and HRS-AKI, the latter being associated with an extremely poor prognosis The American Association for the Study of Liver Disease (AASLD) revised the diagnostic criteria for HRS in June 2021 and recommend prompt treatment as a means of improving outcomes and reducing mortality rates.[3]

Cirrhosis

Cirrhosis is defined as the formation of fibrosis/scarring of the liver secondary to damage caused by various diseases such as Viral Hepatitis, alcohol use, and most commonly nonalcoholic fatty liver disease. As a part of the disease process of cirrhosis, fibrotic tissue replaces normal functioning liver cells and tissue with injured, scarred liver tissue that results in various sized nodules that impair the function of the liver. Cirrhosis is the result of exposure to persistent toxins, both environmental and social that lead to and result in liver failure and possibly death. The resulting liver damage is caused by attempts of the liver to repair itself; however, cirrhotic changes in the liver are irreversible. Excessive consumption of alcohol and steatosis, "fatty liver" are the most significant causative factors in the HRS development (**Fig. 1**). There are 2 types of Cirrhosis, compensated and decompensated.

Decompensated cirrhosis

Decompensated Cirrhosis is the more severe form as complications such as the development of ascites, variceal bleeding, and hepatic encephalopathy, all life-threatening complications that may impair not only an individual's liver health but both an individual's physical and functional health and abilities.[4] In decompensated cirrhosis, nitric oxide combined with additional mediators of vasoactivity cause prolonged vasodilatation, in both the systemic and splenic systems.[4] This process causes a hyperdynamic state that results in an increase in the workload of the heart and impairs/decreases systemic vascular resistance. When the splenic circulatory system functions properly it receives more than 25% of the cardiac output and contains approximately 25% of total blood volume. Splanchnic circulation can, therefore, serve a means to regulate both increased cardiac output distribution as well as a blood reservoir.[5] There are various mechanisms that are involved in splenic circulation including blood volume from the liver and intestines each providing between 300 and 400 mL of the blood.[4,6] Therefore, the splanchnic vasculature serves as an important blood reservoir for the circulatory system. These changes in the circulatory system result in various syndromes including cirrhotic cardiomyopathy.[4,6]

Epidemiology and prevalence of cirrhosis

Cirrhosis is the ninth leading cause of death in the United State. The condition accounts for an estimated 1.2% of all deaths in the United States.[7] Excessive alcohol consumption is the leading preventable cause of death that results in liver damage, and is more common in men, than women. More women die from excessive alcohol use with greater than half of alcohol-attributable deaths resulting from excessive

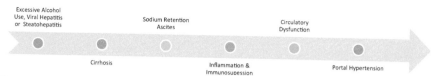

Fig. 1. The sequela of cirrhosis.[4]

alcohol use (defined as greater than 2 alcoholic beverages daily for women and 3 alcoholic beverages daily for men) which over time, can result in Cirrhosis, Steatohepatitis and eventually HRS.[7]

Complication of Cirrhosis

Portal hypertension

PHTN causes gross pressure on the portal vessels, resulting in the secretion of vasodilators, specifically nitric oxide, carbon monoxide, prostacyclins, and endocannabinoids. This causes splanchnic vasodilation and reduced intrahepatic blood volume resulting in a decreased mean arterial blood pressure (MAP). This reduction in the MAP activates both the sympathetic nervous system and the renin–angiotensin–aldosterone system causing the retention of sodium and water. PHTN causes increased abdominal pressure which results in vascular resistance. As a consequence, the blood coming from the portal vein may start to back up, leading to PHTN, which refers to increased blood pressure in the portal vein. As a result, fluid may start to leak out of the portal vein and into the abdomen, leading to ascites.[2]

Ascites. Ascites is defined as a collection of excess fluid in the abdominal cavity that occurs secondary to cirrhosis. When the liver is functioning normally, the liver receives blood from the spleen and gastrointestinal organs through the portal vein. Fibrosis impairs this process resulting in increased abdominal pressure and ascites, which occurs in the late stages of ESRD.[4] The excessive fluid may lead to multiple complication, pulmonary hypertension, heart failure, hepatocellular carcinoma, pancreatitis, and pulmonary tuberculosis.[6,8]

Pathophysiology

The pathophysiologic process of HRS includes a complex myriad of inflammatory, circulatory, and hemodynamic factors. Vasoconstriction of the arteries is the major inciting factor in the myriad that begins with cirrhosis or liver failure that leads to renal dysfunction. The 2 types of HRS have grossly different etiologies but share some similar features. particularly the acute versus chronic presentation of these factors.

The vascular system, cardiovascular dysfunction in addition to hemodynamic changes, and the systemic inflammatory response contribute significantly to this process. All these abnormalities result in factors contributing to HRS. Cytokines are a major factor in HRS that initiates the process. Multiple studies have investigated how liver failure potentiates kidney failure with the common finding being gross systemic inflammation, both vasoconstriction and vasodilation with a rise in serum creatinine (SCr). The new criteria for recognizing HRS are presented in **Table 1**.

Circulatory dysfunction

Cirrhosis results in elevated intrahepatic vascular resistance with splanchnic vasodilatation due to sodium retention, which leads to the development of ascites, and renal impairment. The sequela of cirrhosis results in elevated intrahepatic vascular resistance and splanchnic vasodilatation secondary to AKI according to the International Club of Ascites.[9]

Table 1
Updated guidelines for the diagnosis of hepatorenal syndrome[3,9]

Syndrome	Definition	Hallmark Signs
HRS-AKD	Patients with Cirrhosis and functional kidney injury that do not meet the criteria for HRS-AKI	• History of chronic kidney disease • Use of medications that may be nephrotoxic, such as angiotensin-converting enzymes inhibitors, angiotensin-receptor blockers, and aminoglycosides (list is not inclusive)
HRS-AKI	Characterized by renal failure that occurs at the late stages of cirrhosis.	• Altered cytokine profile • Systemic inflammation • Vasoconstriction of the arteries I • Hepatic failure with cirrhosis • Hyper dynamic circulation • Cirrhotic cardiomyopathy • Adrenal insufficiency

Systemic inflammation

Systemic inflammation has become a major hallmark of liver cirrhosis in both compensated and decompensated cirrhosis. Low-grade inflammation is frequently seen with compensated cirrhosis.[2] Once liver cirrhosis progresses to a decompensated state, immunosuppression develops as a result of the secretion of inhibitory markers. It is proposed that systemic inflammation has a large role in the process with existing, immunosuppression and promotes the development of severe unusual infections which drives inflammation and organ failures.[6]

Historical perspectives

HRS was first described in 1877 by Fredrich Freicis and Austin Flint who noted oliguria in the presence of ascites without structural, renal damage. This finding was further supported by Fritz, who found that the autopsies of individuals with cirrhosis and renal failure demonstrated that there were no histologic changes in the kidneys of individuals with cirrhosis.[1] This realization allowed for the kidneys of individuals who succumbed to the HRS disease process to serve as organ donors and transplantation of the kidneys of individuals in renal failure.[1] Based on this finding, HRS-AKI was found to have no impact on renal function or structure. One of the most notable and useful strategies to aid and improve outcomes of HRS-AKI has been the establishment of new definition and diagnostic criteria based on the recent HRS-AKI presentation, severity of symptoms, and the likelihood of recovery.[3] The most significant criteria change being the removal of an absolute SCr threshold to diagnose HRS-AKI previously known as HRS-1. Establishment of the revised practice guidelines incorporates the guidance provided by the International Club of Ascites 2015 recommendation that may lead to earlier diagnosis which is proposed to improve mortality and treatment outcomes. The revised criteria are now classified as HRS-AKI and HRS-AKD. Of the 2 forms, HRS-AKI is the more progressive and more common form of HRS, with 7% of cases being diagnosed as such and approximately 25% of cases diagnosed as ARS-AKD.

Guidelines, Definitions, and Hallmarks of Hepatorenal Syndrome

The AASLD updated the definition of HRS with the intent to identify the condition earlier and to initiate prompt treatment with the hopes of improving patient outcomes. Refer to **Table 1**.

Diagnostic criteria

In the year 2021, the AASLD released a new set of diagnostic criteria for HRS-AKI which was developed by a multidisciplinary panel of experts who used the Grading of Recommendations Assessment, Development, and Evaluation (GRADE) system. The GRADE System identifies a clear question that seeks to address how outcome criteria are prioritized (Important versus Critical). Additionally, the GRADE system recognizes and considers factors that can reduce the quality of evidence. These factors include study limitations, inconsistency of results, indirectness of evidence, imprecision, and publication biases.[10] The new criteria for diagnosis of HRS are no longer based on a threshold of the creatinine level but rather the diagnosis is based on subtle SCr changes which can be a reliable method to predict HRS-AKI mortality. HRS type 1 has changed to HRS-AKI. HRS type 2 has changed to HRS Nonacute kidney injury (NAKI), with subgroups that include HRS-AKD and HRS-chronic kidney disease.[11] The changes are in **Table 2**.

The 2021 updates to the diagnostic criteria for HRS-AKI facilitate the earlier diagnosis and initiation of treatment which can improve health outcomes. AKI related to HRS is a life-threatening complication of advanced cirrhosis causing high rates of mortality. Eleven percent of the episodes of AKI in hospitalized patients with cirrhosis are attributed to HRS with approximately 50% of patients hospitalized with acute decompensation of cirrhosis developing AKI during hospitalization.[13] Annually, HRS accounts for 4 billion dollars in health care costs.[14]

HRS is primarily a diagnosis of exclusion.[15] Identification of potential risk factors, underlying conditions, and recognition of the appropriate diagnosis early on is key to initiate the appropriate treatment and improve health outcomes. The initial evaluation should focus on the elimination of potentially reversible causes of AKI such as infectious conditions such as human immunodeficiency virus (HIV), bacterial infections, hepatitis B and C, drugs, toxins, autoimmune conditions, hypovolemic or cardiogenic shock, nephrotoxic agents, malignancy, structural damage to the kidney, and genetic disorders before establishing a diagnosis of HRS.[8] Blood, urine, and ascitic cultures and chest radiograph should be obtained as warranted if infection or spontaneous bacterial peritonitis is suspected. For patients with cirrhosis that are not in the advanced stages, evaluation for other potential causes of AKI such as hypovolemia, nephrotoxicity, glomerulonephritis, and acute tubular necrosis (ATN) should be considered. Identification of risk factors that could be contributing to the development of HRS-AKI is also a vital component. Clinical findings that are commonly associated with HRS-AKI include hyponatremia, high plasma renin levels, and severe ascites. Factors that can contribute to the development of HRS-AKI include paracentesis with a large volume of fluid removed with inadequate replacement of albumin and systemic infections that can lead to acute hemodynamic changes. Circulatory dysfunction can occur following paracentesis with a large volume of fluid removed (4.5–5 L or more) causing hypotension, hyponatremia, and a heightened risk for developing HRS-AKI.[6] Administration of albumin following paracentesis is an important intervention that can reduce a patient's risk.

The evaluation and diagnostic work up should include:

- The presence of reduced renal function
- Exclude or treat any underlying conditions that are potentially reversible
- Correct prerenal conditions such as dehydration
- Discontinue any potentially nephrotoxic agents
- Evaluate SCr for an acute rise of 0.3 mL/dL or greater

- Evaluate urinalysis for urinary sediment and urine neutrophil gelatinase-associated lipocalin (NGAL) biomarker (if available)
- Determine stage of AKI
- Manage and treat identified potential risk factors
- Monitor for the improvement of symptoms or continued rise in SCr
- Administer albumin 1 g/kg infusion for 2 days
- Evaluate the patient for improvement or resolution[8]

An acute rise in SCr of 0.3 mg/dl or greater should prompt the evaluation of a urinalysis including urinary sediment and biomarkers to rule out potentially competing diagnoses such as ATN, AKI, urinary tract infections, and urinary tract obstruction.[8] The clinical presentation of HRS-AKI and ATN are very similar which may make differentiating diagnoses difficult. HRS-AKI is characterized by the presence of proteinuria (>500 mg/d), absence of shock, and microhematuria (>50 rbc/hpf), and normal kidney ultrasound.[6] Proteinuria and hematuria can be representative of tubular damage thus ATN cannot be completely excluded. Urinary sediment and presence of urinary NGAL biomarker may be helpful when identifying or eliminating potentially competing diagnosis such as ATN. Replacement of fluid volume is recommended for the treatment of suspected prerenal AKI.[16] Cautious evaluation of cardiopulmonary status is important especially when expanding fluid volume. The accuracy of urinary NGAL results improves following fluid replacement as recommended for the treatment of AKI.[6] A fractional excretion of urinary sodium of less than 1% may be indicating HRS. However, caution should be used when evaluating urine sodium results. Diuretics and the presence of dehydration are examples of factors that can alter urine sodium results.

The management and treatment of risk factors may include addressing underlying conditions, discontinuing nephrotoxic medications or diuretics, treatment of infections, volume replacement, prevention of hypotension, administering albumin following large-volume paracentesis, and treatment of obstructive uropathy.[8] An albumin challenge can be used if the SCr continues to rise despite the treatment of underlying conditions.[8] Improvement or resolutions of symptoms following an albumin challenge is indicative for HRS.[8]

Table 2
New HRS diagnostic criteria[12]

Criteria Prior to 2021	New Criteria 2021
HRS Type 1 • Serum creatinine doubles >2.5 mg/dL in 2 wk	HRS-AKI • Increase in serum creatinine of 0.3 mg/dL within 48 h or • Serum creatinine increases by 1.5 times that of baseline level (3 mo prior)
HRS Type 2 • Gradual increase in creatinine level not meeting criteria above	HRS-NAKI • HRS AKD Estimated glomerular filtration rate of < 60 mL/min for <3 mo without any other signs of kidney disease or <50% increase in serum creatinine from baseline level (3 mo prior) • HRS CKD Estimated glomerular filtration rate of < 60 mL/min for >3 mo without any other signs of kidney disease

Management and Treatment

Prevention and treatment of precipitant factors that can contribute to worsening kidney function is an important component of the management and treatment of HRS-AKI. Hypovolemia in the presence of cirrhosis should be avoided thus it is important to monitor patients with cirrhosis closely. Approximately 90% of prerenal AKI stage 1 resolves with fluid replacement.[6] Treatment is dependent on baseline level of liver and kidney function and early recognition of AKI and HRS. During hospitalization, strategies to prevent the decompensation of advanced cirrhosis are crucial. Nephrotoxic agents should be avoided to reduce the risk for the development of AKI. Current medication regimens should be closely monitored to reduce the risk for nephrotoxicity. Maintaining appropriate hydration and hemodynamic status will prevent cardiopulmonary compromise and reduced kidney perfusion.

On diagnosis of HRS-AKI an albumin challenge should be initiated with albumin 20% to 25% at a dose of 1 g per kilogram per day for 2 days.[6,8] Diuretics should be discontinued during albumin infusion to avoid further volume depletion.[6] Prophylactic antibiotics should be used following a variceal bleed, infection, and for the prevention of spontaneous bacterial peritonitis.[14] Approximately 30% of patients with bacterial peritonitis develop HRS-AKI.[6] Intravenous albumin should be administered for patients having a large-volume paracentesis and with spontaneous bacterial peritonitis (1.5 g/kg for one dose followed by 1 g/kg on day 3).[14] Evidence has demonstrated that the incidence of hepatorenal syndrome, spontaneous bacterial peritonitis, and mortality decreases with the administration of intravenous albumin.[14]

Vasoconstrictive agents such as terlipressin, a synthetic vasopressin analog with selective vasopressin 1 activity, or norepinephrine may be used in combination with albumin for patients with HRS-AKI to improve kidney function.[6,8] Vasoconstrictive agents and albumin are often used for patients with AKI Stage 1B or higher. Reversal of HRS can occur with the concomitant use of vasoconstrictors and albumin infusion. Splanchnic vasoconstriction in patients with cirrhosis will decrease intraabdominal pressure caused by ascites and improve renal blood flow.[6] Studies have demonstrated that the use of terlipressin and albumin for the treatment of HRS can lead to a 20% to 80% improvement.[6,14] Fewer studies are currently available evaluating the effects of norepinephrine to treat HRS-AKI; however, results seem to be similar to terlipressin.[8] Vasoconstrictor agents are used until the SCr returns to baseline levels which may take up to 14 days or longer. Some patients may require longer treatment to prevent recurrent HRS-AKI.[8] Forty to 50 g of albumin can be infused daily in conjunction with vasoconstrictive agents for continued therapy if indicated.[8] It is important to note that despite the proven efficacy of terlipressin at this time it has not yet been approved for use in the United States for the treatment of HRS-AKI.[8] Serious side effects of terlipressin include cardiovascular risks such as pulmonary edema, myocardial infarction, ischemia of the fingers or toes, and mesenteric ischemia.[14] Cautious monitoring of fluid volume status and for ischemic effects should occur at least twice a day when terlipressin is used. Administering terlipressin via continuous infusion may reduce the risk for ischemic side effects.[8] It is also important to evaluate cardiac risk, baseline liver and renal function before initiating treatment with terlipressin.[14] Terlipressin should be avoided in patients with a history of coronary artery disease and/or peripheral vascular disease. Norepinephrine 0.5 mg per hour is administered via continuous infusion to a maximum of 3 mg per hour as warranted depending on mean arterial pressure.[8] The goal of a norepinephrine infusion is to increase the mean arterial pressure by 10 mm Hg or more and improve the urine output to more than 200 mL of urine within 4 hours.[8] Adverse events related to treatment are less common with the use of norepinephrine.[6] Patients should, however, be monitored for tachy- or bradyarrhythmias. Vasoconstrictors should be discontinued if improvement in the SCr occurs within a week.[17]

The response to treatment is dependent on several factors. More severe liver disease, sepsis, multi-system organ failure, and higher SCr levels before initiating treatment can negatively impact the response to treatment. Lower SCr levels are associated with higher rates of reversal of HRS.[6]

Renal replacement therapies can be considered depending on the severity of the patient's condition, and the ability to maintain acid–base and electrolyte balance with medical management. If fluid volume, electrolyte, and acid–base disturbances are not responding to medical management, renal replacement therapies may be used. Intermittent hemodialysis may be used to treat azotemia, electrolyte, and acid–base disturbances if the patient is hemodynamically stable. Continuous renal replacement therapy (CRRT) may be used to treat azotemia, electrolyte, and acid–base disturbances in the presence of higher risk for cardiovascular compromise.

When feasible, liver transplantation is the best treatment option for HRS that results in permanent dysfunction despite treatment. Recovery of kidney function may not occur following liver transplant and is dependent on factors such as the duration of AKI and preexisting underlying chronic comorbid conditions. For the presence of prolonged AKI or presence of end stage renal disease, kidney–liver transplantation is the preferred method for HRS-AKI if possible. To meet the criteria for a liver–kidney transplant, the patient must have sustained AKI, CKD stage 4 (eGFR 20 mL/min or less) for a minimum of 6 weeks. Unfortunately, despite liver–kidney transplant, kidney disease may persist.

SUMMARY

Cirrhosis is a complex disease and has devastating effects on the liver. People living with the condition are at risk for many complications such as HRS. If diagnosed with this condition, the prognosis is often poor. Therefore, it is imperative that treating providers are aware of the symptoms and methods to either prevent or adequately treat the syndrome. Timely referral, prevention, early recognition, and initiation of treatment are key components for prevention or to improve the prognosis for HRS. Excluding potentially contributing factors and/or conditions is also vitally important for diagnostic purposes. Comorbid conditions may be present and further complicate diagnosis. Fluid volume replacement, administration of albumin, and vasoconstrictors as warranted are important for improving the hemodynamic status and potential reversal of HRS-AKI.

CLINICS CARE POINTS

- Cirrhosis is a major factor in the development of hepatorenal syndrome (HRS).
- Early diagnosis of HRS results in a better prognosis.
- Updated guidelines for the diagnosis of HRS do not focus solely on serum creatinine (SCr).
- Prevention and treatment of precipitant factors that can contribute to worsening kidney function is an important component of the management and treatment of HRS-acute kidney injury (HRS-AKI).
- Vasoconstrictive agents such as terlipressin or norepinephrine may be used in combination with albumin for patients with HRS-AKI to improve kidney function.

DISCLOSURE

The authors have nothing to disclose.

REFERENCES

1. Ng CKF, Chan MHM, Tai MHI, et al. Hepatorenal syndrome. Clin Biochem 2007; l25:1–17.
2. Hasan I, Rashid T, Chirila RM, et al. Hepatorenal syndrome: pathophysiology and evidence-based management update. Rom J Intern Med 2021;(l59):227–61.
3. Flamm SL, Brown K, Wadei HM, et al. The current management of hepatorenal syndrome–acute kidney injury in the United States and the potential of terlipressin. Liver Transformation 2021;(l8):1191–202.
4. Chandna S, Zarate ER, Gallegos-Orozco JF. Management of decompensated cirrhosis and associated syndromes. Surg Clin North Am 2022;(l102):117–37.
5. Zhang X, Schiano TD, Doyle E, et al. A comparative study of cirrhosis sub-staging using Laennec system, Beijing classification, and morphometry. Mod Pathol 2021;(l34):2175–82.
6. Simonetto DA, Gines P, Kamath PS. Hepatorenal syndrome: pathophysiology, diagnosis, and management. Br Med J 2020;(l370):1–15.
7. Centers for disease control and prevention, health statistics. 2021. Available at: https://www.cdc.gov/nchs/fastats/liver-disease.htm. Accessed February 8, 2022.
8. Biggins SW, Angeli P, Garcia-Tsao G, et al. Diagnosis, evaluation, and management of ascites. Association for the study of liver diseases. Hepatology 2021; 74:1014–48.
9. Angeli P, Ginès P, Wong F, et al. Diagnosis and management of acute kidney injury in patients with cirrhosis: revised consensus recommendations of the International Club of Ascites. Gut 2015;(l64):531–7.
10. Kavanaugh BP. The GRADE system for rating clinical guidelines. PLoS Med 2009; l6(9):1–5.
11. Wong F, Pappas SC, Vargas HE, et al. April 10–14, 2019 The diagnosis of hepatorenal syndrome (HRS): how much does use of the 2015 revised consensus recommendations affect earlier treatment and serum creatinine (SCr) at treatment start? Poster presented at: International Liver Congress™ of the European Association for the Study of the Liver; Vienna, Austria. Poster SAT-141.
12. Angeli P, Garcia-Tsao G,N, Nadim MK, et al. News in pathophysiology, definition and classification of hepatorenal syndrome: a step beyond the International Club of Ascites consensus document. J Hepatol 2019;(l4):811–22.
13. Amin AA, Alabsawy EI, Jalan R, et al. Epidemiology, pathophysiology, and management of hepatorenal syndrome. Semin Nephrol 2019;(l39–1):17–30.
14. Francoz C, Durand F, Kahn J, et al. Hepatorenal syndrome. Clin J Am Soc Nephrol 2019;(l14):774–81.
15. Ojeda-Yuren AS, Cerda-Reyes E, Herrero-Maceda MR, et al. An integrated review of the hepatorenal syndrome. Ann Hepatol 2021;(l22):1–6.
16. de Carvalho JR, Villela-Nogueira CA, Luiz RR, et al. Acute kidney injury network criteria as a predictor of hospital mortality in cirrhotic patients with ascites. J Clin Gastroenterol 2012;l46:e21–6.
17. Khemichian S, Francoz C, Durand F, et al. Hepatorenal syndrome. Crit Care Clin 2021;(l37):321–34.

Hepatic Encephalopathy
Diagnosis and Treatment in Advanced Liver Disease

Vickie Reed, DNP, APRN-NP, C

KEYWORDS

- Hepatic encephalopathy • Acute liver failure • Rifaximin • Portal hypertension
- Hyperammonemia • Neuronal dysfunction • Portosystemic shunting
- Decompensation

KEY POINTS

- Hepatic encephalopathy is a major complication of advanced liver disease.
- Eighty percent of individuals with cirrhosis have minimal covert hepatic encephalopathy.
- Medical guidelines are targeted to individuals with cirrhosis and overt hepatic encephalopathy.
- Hepatic encephalopathy is categorized according to the West Haven Criteria and InternationalSociety for Hepatic Encephalopathy and Nitrogen Metabolism.
- Hepatic encephalopathy is classified by underlying disease, severity, time course, and precipitating factors.

INTRODUCTION

According to data from the CDC's National Center for Health Statistics, chronic liver disease and cirrhosis affect approximately 45.5 million Americans.[1-3] HE, jaundice, ascites, and hepatorenal syndrome are the most researched complications resulting from chronic liver disease. The presence of these clinical disorders in the setting of liver disease is a precursor for increase in morbidity and mortality for those in this group.

Alone, HE is a symptom of progressive advanced liver disease. HE, when associated with liver disease, is a neuropsychiatric abnormality that causes deterioration in cognition, sleep cycle, memory, and fine motor skills.[4] This manifestation of liver disease can be minimally present or overt with signs of confusion. At any measure of HE, it is a precursor for declining quality of life, increased use of health care dollars, and incidence of death. Early recognition of HE provides an opportunity to prevent or

Veterans Health Administration, North-Western Iowa VAMC, 4101 Woolworth Ave, Medicine Dept 111, Omaha, NE 68105, USA
E-mail address: Vickie.Reed@va.gov

Crit Care Nurs Clin N Am 34 (2022) 331–339
https://doi.org/10.1016/j.cnc.2022.04.011
0899-5885/22/Published by Elsevier Inc.

reduce admissions occurring from overt neuropsychiatric complications associated with HE. Outcome prediction is crucial in assisting clinicians' decision-making and allocating limited medical resources.[5]

Development of cirrhosis related complications such as ascites, gastrointestinal bleeding, and HE mark the transition from stable compensated to decompensated liver disease.[6] Studies have shown that in patients with cirrhosis who develop HE, the 1-year and 3-year survival rate are 42% and 23%, respectively.[7,8] Individuals with higher grade overt HE have even greater risk of liver transplant wait-list mortality and lower 1-year and 5-year survival rates after liver transplant.[9–11] In a retrospective study by Peeraphadit and colleagues,[11] of 830 consecutive patients with cirrhosis at 90 days after initial intensive care unit (ICU) admission, 280 patients (33.9%) had died. This study acknowledge that the deceased patients were more likely to have HE, hepatorenal syndrome, spontaneous bacterial peritonitis, acute kidney injury, cardiogenic shock, and septic shock.

HE is not one specific disease but is a term to describe various reversible neuropsychiatric symptoms related to liver dysfunction and/or portosystemic shunting. Identifying HE is often complicated when presented in alcohol use disorder and can become even more complicated when the underlying cause is associated with neurologic manifestations such as alcoholic liver disease or Wilson disease. Therefore, it is important to perform a focused history and physical examination that eliminates other neurologic causes leaving liver disease as the precipitating factor.

Once HE related to advanced liver disease and cirrhosis is identified as the most likely cause, clinical efforts advance to categorizing and grading the degree of HE. Distinguishing HE in the setting of acute liver failure in comparison to long-term existing cirrhosis guides decisions on prognosis and treatment options. Understanding the possible pathogenesis pathways of cirrhosis is multifactorial but necessary to identify onset and select treatment options.

DEFINITION: WHAT IS HEPATIC ENCEPHALOPATHY

According to the AASLD and EASL 2014 practice guidelines, there are many hypotheses on the pathogenesis of HE. The AASLD and EASL define hepatic encephalopathy as a brain dysfunction caused by liver insufficiency and/or portosystemic shunting. Therefore, the purpose of the AASLD and EASL guidelines is to provide standardized terminology and recommendations to all health care workers who have patients with HE, regardless of their medical discipline.[12] There are several suspected pathways leading to disruption in ammonia metabolism that can lead to HE, but ammonia levels are not the mainstay for diagnosing HE. Although the pathway to HE is not clearly understood, it is thought to include hyperammonemia, alterations in gut microbiota, inflammation, and changes in expression and activation of neurotransmitters.[6] Disorders in these pathways can occur simultaneously, making it necessary for the clinician to perform a careful neurologic examination, as no specific laboratory or imaging test is used to conclusively diagnose HE.

PATHOGENESIS OF HEPATIC ENCEPHALOPATHY

For purposes of this article, the exact pathogenesis in the development of HE is yet to be determined and is not implied.[13] Most reviews of literature emphasize on the known normal activity in contrast to the changes associated with advanced liver disease. Such changes are reflected in the increased production of neurotoxins, impairment of neurotransmission, systemic inflammation, alteration of the blood-brain barrier, and alterations in energy metabolism. Further due diligence in review of clinical research and application are warranted. This review provides a minimal overview of neurotoxins in the development of HE.

Normal Function

- Ammonia (NH3) is a nitrogenous toxin produced by bacterial catabolism of urea in the colon.
- NH3 is metabolized in the liver.
- NH3 is cleared by the kidneys and muscles.

Liver Failure

- NH3 is shunted to the systemic circulation instead of metabolized in the liver.
- NH3 crosses the blood-brain barrier and is metabolized in the astrocytes to glutamine.
- Glutamine leads to astrocyte swelling and formation of reactive oxygen species, resulting in brain swelling causing HE.
- NH3 creates inactivation of neuronal chloride extrusion pumps and increases the resting membrane potential.
- Inhibiting postsynaptic potential formation and depolarizing neurons.
- Glutaminase haplotypes are associated with mitochondrial NH3, worsening brain swelling (**Fig. 1, Table 1**).

CLINICAL MANIFESTATIONS

HE manifests as a wide spectrum of neurologic and/or psychiatric abnormalities ranging from subclinical alterations to coma. Individuals exhibiting symptoms of HE will show negative changes in behavior, cognition, and motor system functions.[4,12] The severity of HE will guide the clinician in determining the prognosis and course of treatment.

Clinical Presentation: Physical Manifestations of Advanced Liver Disease

Asterixis (flapping tremor)
Disorientation
Falls
Motor Vehicle Accidents
Muscle wasting
Loss of working memory
Impairments in sleep
Tremors
Personality changes
Irritability
Disinhibition

DIAGNOSIS CLASSIFICATION

There are 4 main factors identified by the AASLD/EASL practice guidelines classifying the severity of HE. The classification system aims to identify (1) the cause, (2) severity of disease, (3) timeline, and (4) precipitating factors of the underlying disease.[12] HE is further divided according to the International Society for Hepatic Encephalopathy and Nitrogen Metabolism (ISHEN) distinction between minimal (covert) and obvious (overt) encephalopathy presentation, with the onset of disorientation or asterixis identifying the onset of overt HE.[4,12]

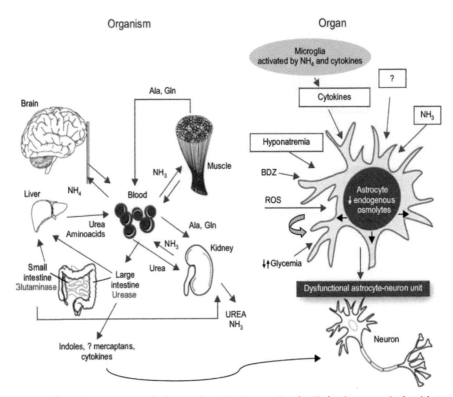

Fig. 1. Effects of Ammonia Imbalances. (Lee SS, Moreau R, eds. Cirrhosis: a practical guide to management. Chichester: John Wiley & Sons, 2015.)

Within the underlying disease classification, HE is subdivided into types A, B, and C. Type A resulting from acute liver failure, type B from portosystemic bypass or shunting, and type C from cirrhosis. The severity grading refers to functional impairments described by the West Haven Criteria and ISHEN classification systems. The course of disease is further categorized into episodic, recurrent, and persistent, referring to the number of episodes over a period of time. Lastly, precipitating factors are complications associated with overt HE type C and should be identified and treated. The most common precipitating factors in episodic HE are infections, which include spontaneous bacterial peritonitis, urinary tract infections, respiratory infections, skin infections, and sepsis.[12] When categorizing HE in a patient, one description from each of the classifications—type, grade, time course, and precipitating factors—should be noted (**Fig. 2**; see **Fig. 4**).

PRECIPITATING FACTORS OF HEPATIC ENCEPHALOPATHY

Hyponatremia
Acid base disturbances
Medication noncompliance
Infection
Gastrointestinal bleeding
Sedating medications
Hypoxia

Table 1
Ammonia to blood-brain barrier[4,7,13]

	Normal Liver Function	Advanced Liver Disease
Liver	Metabolizes ammonia, converting ammonia to urea, preventing entry to systemic circulation	Reduced capacity to remove ammonia. Damaged hepatocytes & portosystemic shunting causing liver bypass into systemic circulation
Muscle	Low glutamine synthetase activity. Mild NH3 clearing via muscles	Conversion of ammonia to glutamine
Kidney	Ammonia that has been converted to urea is excreted	Excess glutamine. Increased renal ammonia production
Intestine	Produces NH3 by bacterial catabolism of urea in the colon. NH3 is by-product of gut metabolism	Increase in pathogenic gut bacteria and reduction in commensal bacteria

Constipation
Spontaneous portosystemic shunts

A specific process or test for HE is difficult to identify because of the multidimensional dysfunction of HE. There are several cognitive, psychophysiological tools that can be used in evaluating individuals with suspected HE. These tests have interobserver variability and often require trained examiners. The most difficult to diagnose is the covert HE (CHE). However, it is important to identify CHE, as this is a precursor of overt hepatic encephalopathy (OHE) leading to poor quality of life and recurrent hospitalizations. An operational approach may be to test patients who have problems with their quality of life or in whom there are complaints from the patients and their relatives.[12] Suraweera and colleagues[14–16] have a diagnostic and treatment algorithm noted in **Fig. 3**.

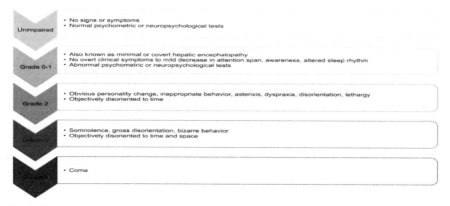

Fig. 2. West Haven Criteria Classification of Hepatic Encephalopathy. (*Referenced from* Suraweera, D., Sundaram, V., & Saab, S. Evaluation and Management of Hepatic Encephalopathy: Current Status and Future Directions. Gut and Liver, 2016, 10(4), 509-519. This is an Open Access article distributed under the terms of the Creative Commons Attribution Non-Commercial License (http://creativecommons.org/licenses/by-nc/4.0) which permits unrestricted non-commercial use, distribution, and reproduction in any medium, provided the original work is properly cited.)

TEST FOR COVERT HEPATIC ENCEPHALOPATHY

Portosystemic encephalopathy
The Critical Flicker Frequency
The Continuous Reaction Time
The Inhibitory Control Test
The Stroop (EncephalApp)
The SCAN test
Electroencephalography examination

TREATMENT

The most current HE treatment recommendations are noted in the 2014 practice guidelines. Treatment of HE is reserved for OHE, type C. Individuals categorized into type C are those with underlying cirrhosis. Episodes of OHE in type C can be spontaneous or precipitated and/or recurrent. Primary prophylaxis may be necessary if the cirrhotic person is at high risk of developing HE. After a first occurrence of HE, initiation of secondary prophylaxis is recommended. It is likely that precipitating factors are involved in OHE. If so, controlling these factors supersedes direct HE treatment. Nearly 90% of patients can be treated with just correction of precipitating factors.[12] Exclusion of other neurologic dysfunction by clinical, laboratory, and radiological assessment are warranted, as HE is a diagnosis of exclusion (**Fig. 4**).

As much of this topic is shown to be complicated, so are the discussions for medical therapy. Most drugs have not been tested by rigorous randomized controlled studies and are used based on circumstantial observations.[12] The most commonly used drugs belong to the nonabsorbable disaccharides such as lactulose and antimicrobials such as rifaximin.

The first drug recommendation for OHE is the nonabsorbable disaccharide, lactulose. It is prescribed to induce at least 2 bowel movements per day. Lactulose is appreciated not only for its laxative effect but also for the prebiotic and acidifying

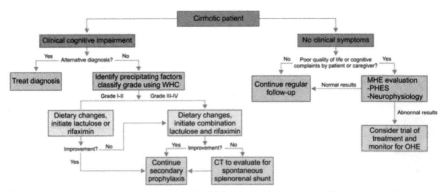

Fig. 3. Evaluation and Management of HE in cirrhotic patients. (*Referenced from* Suraweera, D., Sundaram, V., & Saab, S. Evaluation and Management of Hepatic Encephalopathy: Current Status and Future Directions. Gut and Liver, 2016, 10(4), 509-519. This is an Open Access article distributed under the terms of the Creative Commons Attribution Non-Commercial License (http://creativecommons.org/licenses/by-nc/4.0) which permits unrestricted non-commercial use, distribution, and reproduction in any medium, provided the original work is properly cited.)

Type	Grade			Time Course	Spontaneous or Precipitated
A	MHE	Covert		Episodic	Spontaneous
B	1			Recurrent	
	2				Precipitated (Specify)
C	3	Overt		Persistent	
	4				

Fig. 4. Patients should be characterized by one component from each of the 4 columns. (*Adapted from* Vilstrup et al., Hepatic Encephalopathy in Chronic Liver Disease: 2014 Practice Guideline by the American Association for the Study of Liver Diseases and the European Association for the Study of the Liver, Journal of Hepatology with Permission.)

benefits on the gut metabolism. Lactulose is dosed at 25 mL every 1 to 2 hours until at least 2 soft or loose bowel movements per day are produced; then it is titrated to maintain the 2 to 3 bowel movements per day.[7,12]

Patients with recurrent OHE benefit from the antibiotic, rifaximin, 550 mg, twice a day as an add-on therapy with lactulose. The combination of drugs is effective in preventing recurrent OHE. Krishnarao and Gordon note that rifaximin therapy in conjunction with lactulose use has been shown to significantly reduce the risk of an episode of HE over a 6-month period, and the addition of rifaximin also shows significant reduction in the risk of hospitalization due to HE.[16] There are many other drugs that can be useful in managing OHE; however, studies to support their efficacy are limited. The recent guidelines note that these drugs can safely be used despite their limited proven efficacy.

ADDITIONAL NOVEL HEPATIC ENCEPHALOPATHY THERAPIES

- Branched chain amino acids
- Metabolic ammonia scavengers
- L-ornithine L-aspartate
- Probiotics
- Glutaminase inhibitors
- Neomycin
- Metronidazole
- Flumazenil

DISCUSSION

The occurrence of hepatic encephalopathy is a measure of diminishing quality of life and increased morbidity and mortality. Although overt encephalopathy is the most recognized and treated, minimal hepatic encephalopathy is also an indicator of diminishing quality of life. Treatment of hepatic encephalopathy is reserved for overt HE but may be necessary for those with minimal signs of HE when there is concern from friends and family regarding the individuals cognitive functioning. Classifying HE should involve identification of the type, grade, time of course, and any precipitating factors. Researchers have presented multidimensional pathogenesis process for the development of HE; however, the specific pathology remains unclear. The same is true for the medical management of HE. Continued medical research persists for diagnosis and treatment. At this time the first-line therapies are lactulose and rifaximin.

CASE STUDY

Patient A is a 49-year-old African American man. Brought to the emergency department by his fiancé who reports patient has had significant change in consciousness. Changes started with cold symptoms, fever, cough, and congestion. He is obtunded, frail, and dyspneic. He denies any known prior medical history. He tests positive for COVID 19 and is admitted to the ICU. Abnormal laboratory values include creatine 1.6, white blood cell count 22.0, hemoglobin 10.2, total bilirubin 7.8, aspartate aminotransferase 144 U/L, alanine aminotransferase 78 U/L, alkaline phosphatase 140 U/L, Platelets 130 m/L, and ammonia 40 mcg/dL. Chest radiograph shows bilateral consolidated pneumonia. Record review shows he was admitted 3 months ago with confusion and blood loss anemia related to variceal bleed. He had been diagnosed with cirrhosis related to alcohol use disorder and was discharged on lactulose, carvedilol, spironolactone, and furosemide.

Classify the current presentation.

CLINICS CARE POINTS

- HE is a major complication of advanced liver disease.
- Eighty percent of individuals with cirrhosis have minimal CHE.
- Medical guidelines are targeted to individuals with cirrhosis and overt HE.
- HE is categorized according to the West Haven Criteria and InternationalSociety for Hepatic Encephalopathy and Nitrogen Metabolism.
- HE is classified by underlying disease, severity, time course, and precipitating factors.
- Nonabsorbable disaccharides such as lactulose and antibiotics such as rifaximin are most commonly used in type C, cirrhotic overt HE.

DISCLOSURE

The author has no disclosures.

REFERENCES

1. National Center for Health Statistics. Chronic liver disease and cirrhosis. Fast-Stats - Chronic Liver Disease or Cirrhosis (cdc.gov) . Accessed January 17, 2022.
2. Long L, et al. Impact of Hepatic encephalopathy on clinical characteristics and adverse outcomes in prospective and multicenter cohorts of patients with acute on chronic liver disease. Frontiers in Medicine 2021;8. 709884.
3. Aniruddha P, VanMeter S, Stange J. Prevalence of Hepatic encephalopathy from a commercial medical claims database in the United States. Int J Hepatol 2021; 2021. 8542179.
4. Elsaid M, Rustgi VK. Epidemiology of hepatic encephalopathy. Clin Liver Dis 2020;24:157–74.

5. Peeraphadit, et al. Prognostic value of model for end-stage liver disease score measurements on a daily basis in critically ill patients with cirrhosis. Mayo Clinic Proceedings 2015;90(9):1196–206.

6. Rahimi RS, Brown KA, Flamm SL, et al. Overt hepatic encephalopathy: current pharmacologic treatments and improving clinical outcomes. Am J Med 2021; 134:1330–8.

7. Alsahhar JS, Rahimi RS. Updates on the pathophysiology and therapeutic targets for hepatic encephalopathy. Curr Opin Gastroenterol 2019;35(3):145–54.

8. Alimiirah M, Sadiq O, Gordon SC. Novel therapies in hepatic encephalopathy. Clin Liver Dis 2020;24(2):303–15.

9. Wong RJ, Gish RG, Ahmed A. Hepatic encephalopathy is associated with significantly increased mortality among patients awaiting liver transplantation. Liver 2014;20:1454–61.

10. Wojciech P. Minimal hepatic encephalopathy- diagnosis and treatment. Przeglad Gastroenterologiczny 2021;16(4):311–7.

11. Acharya, et al. QuickStroop, a shortened version of EncephalApp, Detects Covert Hepatic Encephalopathy with similar accuracy within one minute. Clin Gastroenterol Hepatol 2022. In Press.

12. Vilstrup, et al. Hepatic encephalopathy in chronic liver disease: 2014 practice guideline by the American association for the study of liver diseases and the European association for the study of the liver. Hepatology 2014;60(2).

13. Hassouneh R, Bajaj JS. Gut microbiota modulation and fecal transplantation: an overview on innovative strategies for hepatic encephalopathy treatment. J Clin Med 2021;10:330.

14. Jindal A, Jagdish RK. Sarcopenia: Ammonia metabolism and hepatic encephalopathy. Clin Mol Hepatol 2019;25(3):270–9.

15. Suraweera, D., Sundaram, V., & Saab, S. Evaluation and management of hepatic encephalopathy: Current status and future directions. Gut and Liver Jul 10(4): 509-519.

16. Krishnarao A, Gordon FD. Prognosis of hepatic encephalopathy. Clin Liver Dis 2020;24:219–29.

Right-Sided Heart Failure and the Liver

Jillian N. Mauriello, MSN, ARNP-C[a], Michelle M. Straughan, MSN, ARNP-C[b],*

KEYWORDS

- Right-sided heart failure • Heart failure • Liver failure • Hepatic congestion
- Congestive hepatopathy • Cirrhosis • Cardiac cirrhosis

KEY POINTS

- The dual diagnosis of heart failure (HF) and liver disease has prognostic implications.
- Patients with known right-sided HF (RHF) should undergo early screening to evaluate for the presence of liver dysfunction.
- Onset of congestive hepatopathy (CH) can be insidious and patients may be asymptomatic until advanced stages.
- Early identification of underlying causes of RHF is essential in reversing CH.
- A cholestatic pattern of laboratory findings is noted in patients with CH.
- Abdominal Ultrasound, abdominal computed tomography (CT) and magnetic resonance imaging (MRI) all provide useful information for screening for CH and complications; however, no single imaging technique to date distinguishes objectively between congestion and fibrosis.
- Treatment of CH is aimed at the identification of etiology of RHF and guideline-directed medical therapies for HF.

INTRODUCTION

Currently, there are 6.2 million people with heart failure (HF) in the United States with 1 million new HF cases being diagnosed annually.[1] Twenty to 30% of patients with acute HF also have liver dysfunction.[2] The dual diagnoses of chronic heart and liver disease has significant prognostic implications.[3]

The relationship between right-sided HF (RHF) and liver failure dates to 1833 when British anatomist Francis Kiernan coined the phrase "Nutmeg Liver" on the microscopic evaluation of a congested liver (**Fig. 1**).[4] The reference, which is still used today, illustrates the mottled appearance of the liver secondary to the congestion of the

[a] Cardiology, Hunter Holmes McGuire VA Medical Center, 1201 Broad Rock Boulevard, Richmond, VA 23249, USA; [b] Medicine, Gulf Coast Veterans Health Care System, 400 Veterans Avenue, Biloxi, MS 39531, USA
* Corresponding author.
E-mail address: Michelle.Straughan@va.gov
Twitter: Michelle.Straughan@va.gov (M.M.S.)

Crit Care Nurs Clin N Am 34 (2022) 341–350
https://doi.org/10.1016/j.cnc.2022.04.003
0899-5885/22/Published by Elsevier Inc.

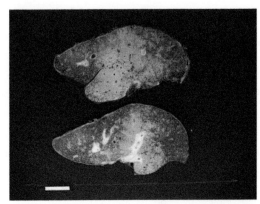

Fig. 1. Nutmeg liver. (*From* Hilscher, M. and Sanchez, W. (2016), Congestive hepatopathy. Clinical Liver Disease, 8: 68-71. https://doi.org/10.1002/cld.573. with permission.)

hepatic vein and leakage of red blood cells from centrilobular sinusoids.[5] By the 1950s, 2 well-known professors in the discipline, Dame Professor Sheila Sherlock and Professor Hans Popper, addressed the liver in cardiac disease through various publications. The clinical cases reflected the common cardiac pathologies at the time; namely rheumatic heart disease with resultant constrictive pericarditis.[6] In the modern era of cardiology; however, ischemic heart disease (IHD) is the predominant cause of HF.

Scrutiny of liver function is primarily driven by evaluation for cardiac transplant candidacy. However, liver disease is often subclinical and underdiagnosed in the early stages of HF.[7] The relationship between the heart and the liver can be classified into 3 categories:

1. liver disease secondary to heart disease
2. heart disease secondary to liver disease
3. systemic diseases that affect both the heart and the liver[8]

The focus of this article will be on liver disease resulting from RHF.

DEFINITIONS

HF is defined as a complex disease that occurs when the ventricle is not able to properly fill or eject blood due to functional or structural impairment.[9]

RHF is a clinical condition for which the right ventricle fails to efficiently pump blood through the pulmonary circulation to meet the demands required for left ventricular filling and systemic circulation.[10]

Congestive hepatopathy (CH) is liver impairment manifested by chronic, passive hepatic venous congestion, impaired hepatic venous outflow secondary to RHF.[8]

Acute cardiogenic liver injury (ACLI) is a complication of low cardiac output and passive congestion which results in significant hypoperfusion to the hepatic system resulting in ischemia and reperfusion injury.[8,11]

BACKGROUND

The primary function of the right ventricle is to return deoxygenated, CO_2-rich blood to the pulmonary vascular system via the pulmonary artery. Thus, allowing for lung perfusion and gas exchange to occur at the alveolar-capillary level. The left ventricle then receives oxygen-rich blood from the pulmonary veins by way of the left atrium which is then pumped through the system for perfusion of the body's organ systems.

The functional and structural differences between the right and left ventricles result in their distinct responses to pressure and volume changes. The right ventricle differs from the left ventricle mainly in that it has a thinner, less muscular wall. Variability in venous return and its larger size makes the right ventricular (RV) more accommodating to abrupt increases in volume, but intolerant to changes in afterload. As opposed to the left ventricle, the right ventricle is more sensitive to abrupt increases in afterload which consequently reduces stroke volume, impairs contractility with subsequent RV dilation.[12]

Mechanisms contributing to the development of RHF are alterations in right-sided filling pressures (preload), increased RV afterload and reduced contractility.[13] Common conditions that cause RHF are left ventricular dysfunction, cardiomyopathy, valvular heart disease, constrictive pericarditis, and congenital heart disease. Cor Pulmonale is the term used to describe RHF secondary to chronic lung diseases such as in pulmonary arterial hypertension (PAH) or chronic obstructive pulmonary disease. In the acute setting, RHF can be caused by RV infarction, pulmonary embolism, or pericardial tamponade.[14]

Hepatic blood flow is dominated by the portal venous system. Compromised forward blood flow in RHF progressively blunts hepatic venous return to the heart resulting in CH.[7] The liver is a resilient organ, capable of preserving its essential functions for an extended period of time. Consequently, early objective signs of liver dysfunction may not be readily apparent. Signs and symptoms of CH often mirror those of RHF, contributing to the delay in diagnosis.[15] Chronic hepatic venous congestion results in cellular hypoxia leading to centrilobular hepatic fibrosis, portal hypertension, and increased risk for hepatocellular carcinoma (HCC). The detrimental hemodynamic consequences of CH may not be evident until significant organ dysfunction has ensued, underscoring the need for clinicians to be aware of the heart–liver axis.[16]

Hepatic impairment is an unavoidable consequence in patients with congenital heart defects who are born with single ventricle physiology. The cardiac Fontan surgery and associated CH is a model for noninflammatory congestive liver disease (**Fig. 2**)[17] The surgery is a considered a palliative measure that prolongs survival and improves the quality of life; however, it is associated with significant liver and renal damage.[17]

Fontan survivors will eventually require a heart transplant. While surgical innovations have increased life expectancy for congenital heart disease, the development of liver failure complicates heart transplant candidacy and future outcomes.[7]

DISCUSSION

CH is a liver disorder arising from chronically elevated central venous pressure, commonly implicated by RHF. It is characterized by diverse hemodynamic and histopathological alterations that fluctuate in conjunction with the clinical course of the underlying cardiac disease[8] The diagnosis of CH is associated with an increased risk for morbidity and mortality, which warrants investigation for liver disease in patients presenting with RHF. CH can eventually progress to cirrhosis, portal hypertension, HCC, acute ischemic hepatitis, and fulminant hepatic failure.[5,8] Disease onset is insidious and often asymptomatic until advanced stages. Laboratory values and imaging do not consistently correlate with the severity of liver impairment or predict long-term outcomes in patients with CH. Serum biomarkers for liver disease are often normal or only

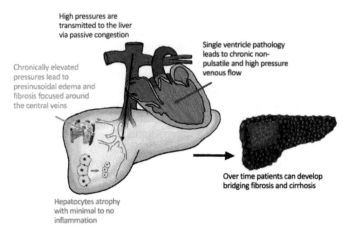

High pressures are transmitted to the liver via passive congestion

Single ventricle pathology leads to chronic non-pulsatile and high pressure venous flow

Chronically elevated pressures lead to presinusoidal edema and fibrosis focused around the central veins

Over time patients can develop bridging fibrosis and cirrhosis

Hepatocytes atrophy with minimal to no inflammation

Fig. 2. Pathophysiology of hepatic congestion in patient with Fontan procedure. (*From* Lemmer A, VanWagner L, Ganger D. Congestive hepatopathy: Differentiating congestion from fibrosis. *Clin Liver Dis (Hoboken)*. 2018;10(6):139-143. Published 2018 Jan 2. https://doi.org/10.1002/cld.676 with permission.)

mildly elevated. Radiographic imaging may be misleading as the nodular appearance of the congested liver can mimic nodules of HCC.[8] Moreover, CH must be differentiated from noncardiac, inflammatory causes of liver damage such as viral hepatitis, fatty liver disease, and autoimmune hepatitis.[17] Consultation with gastroenterology/hepatology specialist is advised when the etiology of liver disease is unclear.

As in HF, hepatic failure causes the activation of the renin–angiotensin–aldosterone system by the kidney due to reduced renal perfusion. Decreased albumin and oncotic pressure in hepatic failure causes interstitial fluid retention Aldosterone secretion in combination with reduced oncotic pressure results in inappropriate water retention, exacerbating the degree of volume overload in HF.[18]

APPROACH

The clinical approach to the management of RHF is focused on preventing clinical decompensation. Identification of the underlying etiology of the disease is essential to forming an individualized treatment strategy. Comprehensive evaluation of the patient's medical history, clinical presentation, and supporting diagnostic data are essential elements used to establish disease pathology.[13] Hemodynamic stability will determine the level of care required. Patients with chronic RHF who are considered stable and well-compensated can be treated on an outpatient basis, whereas patients presenting with acute, decompensated RHF require admission to the intensive care unit.[10] Beyond HF management provided by cardiology, consultation with pulmonology, hepatology, and nephrology providers should be coordinated as clinically indicated based on patient-specific needs.

Guideline-directed medical therapy for HF is the cornerstone of treatment; however, caution should be exercised with the use of antihypertensive agents. Systemic hypotension impairs RV stroke volume and can lead to hemodynamic instability.[12] Correction of volume overload is imperative, yet it is equally important to maintain adequate levels of circulatory volume due to preload dependence in RHF. Diuresis may require inotropic support to maintain cardiac output and end-organ perfusion.[14] Advanced therapies for RHF are inhaled nitric oxide, phophodiasterase5 inhibitors for pulmonary hypertension, hemodynamic support with inotropes, vasopressors, and mechanical ventilation, ventricular assist devices and cardiac transplant.[13]

There is no specific treatment of CH per se. Management is aimed at treating the RHF. Recovery of liver function is observed after relief of the underlying congestion.[17] Impaired hepatic blood flow in the liver affects the function of downstream organs. The kidney responds by the activation of the renin–angiotensin–aldosterone system. The effect of aldosterone leads to inappropriate water retention and hyponatremia. Therefore, the use of an aldosterone antagonist in combination with a loop diuretic is more effective than a loop diuretic alone for better control of peripheral edema and ascites.[18] Spironolactone and eplerenone are examples of aldosterone antagonists. Hyperkalemia and renal failure are possible adverse side effects of this drug class and therefore must be closely monitored upon initiation and throughout the duration of use.

Restriction of sodium and fluid intake is indicated to prevent fluid retention in CH in patients with hyponatremia. Special considerations must be taken to avoid hypotension and hypoxia to ensure adequate hepatic perfusion. Hepatotoxic medications and alcohol intake should be avoided.[5]

CLINICAL EXAMINATION

Patients with RHF and concomitant liver failure can present with symptoms of RHF: fatigue, dry cough, shortness of breath, orthopnea, excessive weight gain, dependent pitting edema, poor appetite, nausea, vomiting, and right upper quadrant pain. Stretching of the Glisson's capsule can cause dull pain in the right upper quadrant of the abdomen.[16] Classic physical examination findings are jugular venous distention, positive hepatojugular reflux, hepatosplenomegaly, ascites, murmur of tricuspid regurgitation and a loud P2 sound associated with pulmonary hypertension.[14]

LABORATORY FINDINGS

Laboratory abnormalities in RHF typically reveal disease acuity and multisystem organ involvement. Elevated brain natriuretic peptide (BNP) is a sensitive indicator of acute HF in patients with clinical symptoms of volume overload, but can also be elevated in other conditions such as tachycardia and renal failure. It is also important to note that BNP may be underestimated in HF patients with obesity.[2] Reduced glomerular filtration rate (GFR), elevated creatinine and cystatin C levels, and anemia of chronic disease are markers of renal impairment, and can be observed in the setting of cardiorenal syndrome, volume overload or dehydration from over diuresis.[2] Electrolyte disturbances are common in HF, and should be monitored closely. This is especially important in patients on diuretic therapy. Liver biochemical markers may reveal elevated bilirubin, normal or mild increase in aminotransferase level, and hypoalbuminemia. Other laboratory findings suggestive of liver dysfunction include anemia, thrombocytopenia, and elevated PT/INR.[14]

Clinical correlation of CH with serum biomarkers is limited, but does provide supporting data in context with clinical findings. Albumin may be mildly decreased; however, this is an unreliable marker as hypoalbuminemia can be secondary to cardiac cachexia resulting from end-stage HF. Prothrombin time (PT) can also be increased but lacks specificity in patients on anticoagulation therapy. Levels of alanine transaminase (ALT) and aspartate aminotransferase (AST) are poor predictors of liver damage and fibrosis in CH.[11] The most notable laboratory abnormalities in CH are alkaline phosphatase (AP), gamma-glutamyl transferase (GGT) and bilirubin. Elevated AP and GGT are markers of cholestasis which reflect impaired drainage of bile into the portal venous system caused by compression of bile ducts by congested hepatic sinusoids.[8] Serum biomarkers of cholestasis in CH have also been found to correspond with right-sided filling pressures clinical volume overload, a provocative concept with future implications for the management of RHF.[3] Elevated bilirubin is a prognostic indicator for worsening outcomes in patients with pulmonary hypertension and is a strong predictor of all-cause mortality in patients with HF.[6,14]

Ascites should be evaluated with diagnostic paracentesis to determine whether the etiology is cardiac or cirrhotic. Cardiac and cirrhotic ascites both demonstrate elevated serum-ascites albumin gradient. However, cardiac ascites will contain higher protein levels (>2.5 g/dL), LDH, and red blood cells.[8]

DIAGNOSTICS

Electrocardiogram may reveal RV hypertrophy, right bundle branch block, or atrial arrhythmias. Patterns of RV strain can be seen in acute pulmonary embolism.

Echocardiography is performed to evaluate overall cardiac structure & function. Information obtained is valuable in determining the degree of RHF and the underlying cause. RV systolic function is calculated by the measurement of tricuspid annular plane systolic excursion (TAPSE). Reduced RV systolic function, RV dilation, RV hypertrophy, and right atrial enlargement are possible finding in RHF. The etiology of RHF may be identified by the presence of underlying valvulopathy, left ventricular dysfunction if there is reduced left ventricular ejection fraction, or elevated pulmonary pressures suggesting PAH.[13]

Cardiac MRI is a valuable tool for the assessment of cardiac morphology, structure, and function. This is helpful if insufficient data is obtained by echocardiogram due to poor imaging windows. Cardiac MRI provides advanced imaging for the diagnosis of specific cardiomyopathies.

Cardiac catheterization is the gold standard for definitive diagnosis of RHF and its etiology. Combined right and left heart catheterization provides the most comprehensive evaluation. In addition to the assessment and quantification of valvular heart disease, right heart catheterization provides precise measurements of right and left-sided filling pressures, pulmonary arterial pressures, and cardiac output. The role of left heart catheterization is diagnostic and therapeutic. The primary indication for this procedure is the evaluation of the coronary arteries and stenting of obstructive coronary lesions. Simultaneously, cardiac output is measured and the severity of left-sided valvulopathies can be assessed.

When attempting to distinguish between liver fibrosis or congestion, no imaging modality provides a clear distinction between the 2.[17] However, imaging is useful in supporting a diagnosis of CH and screening for complications (**Table 1**).[8] Abdominal ultrasound is generally the initial modality selected for the evaluation of the liver and it provides information related to hepatic structure and blood flow. Computed tomography (CT), and magnetic resonance imaging (MRI) with intravenous contrast enhancement provides a more detailed view of the liver and surrounding structures as well as the function of the liver.[8] Fibroscan, also known as transient elastography, is a useful noninvasive modality for assessing stiffness in scarring in liver fibrosis, its utility in evaluating congestion hepatopathy is less appreciated.[17]

The model for end-stage liver disease (MELD) score is a tool that is useful in risk stratifying for postoperative complications in orthotopic heart transplant recipients.[7] The MELD score factors in serum creatinine, bilirubin, PT, and sodium into a scoring system. Patients with high modified meld scores (which exclude PT in patients on chronic anticoagulation) are at risk for intraoperative events to include postoperative

Table 1
Imaging modalities

Imaging study	Identifies	Results
Transabdominal Ultrasound	Liver size and structure, blood flow and pressures in the portal system	Hepatomegaly, dilated IVC and hepatic veins, nodular appearance of liver,
Abdominal CT scan/MRI	Liver size structure and morphology	Hepatomegaly, nodular appearance of liver, Focal nodular hyperplasia (FNH) washout appearance, mimics HCC

Data from "Lemmer A, VanWagner L, Ganger D. Congestive hepatopathy: Differentiating congestion from fibrosis. *Clin Liver Dis (Hoboken)*. 2018;10(6):139-143. Published 2018 Jan 2. doi:10.1002/cld.676."

bleeding, renal failure, and in hospital death.[7] However, MELD score is not a useful tool to predict risk for decompensation in CH.[17]

CONSIDERATIONS

Management of patients with RHF and liver failure requires a collaborative approach led by advanced HF and hepatology specialists. Collaboration with other specialty providers in pulmonology, nephrology, surgery, interventional cardiology, and radiology is commonly required to tailor an individualized treatment plan. The interdisciplinary team should include an expert team of physicians, nurses, and pharmacists in a medical center whereby complex diagnostic tests and imaging can be performed and accurately interpreted. Collegial rapport between inpatient and outpatient providers of all specialties is vital to ensure continuity of high quality, safe and effective care.

Patients with end-stage HF may be referred for cardiac transplant or left ventricular assist device (LVAD) and in some cases, these measures may help improve CH.[5] Patients considered for cardiac transplantation who have elevated markers of cholestasis may require a liver biopsy to exclude cirrhosis.[14] "Histopathological findings of congestive liver disease include presinusoidal edema, pericellular fibrosis centered around the central veins, and in later-stage disease central-to-central and central-to-portal bridging fibrosis with regenerative nodules. Minimal inflammation is present microscopically because hepatocyte death seems to occur through atrophy and apoptosis."[17] However, liver biopsies may not represent good clinical prediction in liver outcomes following heart transplantation.[17] Consultation with the surgical team is required to determine cardiac transplant candidacy and provide recommendations for the care of transplant recipients or patients with congenital heart surgery.

An additional consideration is screening for HCC in CH. Although there are no guidelines established, a reasonable approach is to perform twice yearly screening in patients with cardiac cirrhosis.

Despite advances in management and novel approaches, HF is a chronic, progressive disease. Medical therapies can slow disease progression, but rarely do they lead to the reversal of HF.[19] In many instances these therapies can prolong the more advanced stages of HF.[19] This, in turn, places a significant burden on health care systems as well as on patients and their caregivers. It is imperative to begin early in shared decision making and goals of care discussions. Palliative care used in conjunction with disease-modifying therapies provides a patient-centered approach to ensure that treatments are in line with patient goals across the continuum of disease progression.

SUMMARY

Advances in medical and surgical therapies for HF have led to increased long-term survival in this population, resulting in a higher incidence of liver complications. Therefore, it is essential for clinicians to understand the dynamic interactions between the heart and liver to provide optimal management of patients with cardio hepatic failure. CH is an ominous complication of RHF which may be overlooked at its initial onset. Evaluation of liver function should be included in the early stages of RHF to assess for evolving hepatopathy.[8] Markers of CH have been found to correspond to the degree of right-sided filling pressures and systemic congestion illustrating the utility of liver function assessment as a prognostic indicator of RHF.[3] Unfortunately, determining the severity and prognosis of liver disease remains a challenge due to limitations in standardized, objective testing modalities specific to CH.[8] Acquisition of novel biomarkers and scoring systems are needed to better risk stratify these patients and to improve prognosis and long-term survival.

CLINICAL PEARLS

- The dual diagnosis of heart failure (HF) and liver disease has prognostic implications
- Patients with known right-sided HF (RHF) should undergo early screening to evaluate for the presence of liver dysfunction
- Onset of congestive hepatopathy (CH) can be insidious and patients may be asymptomatic until advanced stages
- Early identification of underlying causes of RHF is essential in reversing CH
- A cholestatic pattern of laboratory findings is noted in patients with CH
- Abdominal ultrasound, abdominal computed tomography (CT), and magnetic resonance all provide useful information for screening for CH and complications; however, no single imaging technique to date distinguishes objectively between congestion and fibrosis.
- Treatment of CH is aimed at the identification of etiology of RHF and guideline-directed medical therapies for HF

CLINICS CARE POINTS

- Congestive hepatopathy is an ominous complication of right heart failure which may be overlooked at its initial onset.
- Identifictaion of underlying etiology is essential in forming an individualized treatment plan.
- Guideline-directed medical therapy for heart failure is the cornerstone of treatment; however, caution should be exercised with use of antihypertensive agents.Management is aimed at treating the right heart failure.
- Recovery of liver function is observed after relief of the underlying congestion.[17] Management of patients with right heart fialure and liver failure requires a collaborative approach.

ACKNOWLEDGMENTS

The contents do not represent the views of the U.S. Department of Veterans Affairs or the United States Government.

This material is the result of work supported with resources and the use of facilities at the Gulf Coast Veterans Health Care System, Biloxi, Mississippi.

DISCLOSURE

The authors have nothing to disclose.

REFERENCES

1. Bozkurt B, Hershberger RE, Butler J, et al. ACC/AHA Key data elements and Definitions for heart failure: a Report of the American College of cardiology/American heart association Task Force on clinical data standards (Writing Committee to Develop clinical data standards for heart failure). Circ Cardiovasc Qual Outcomes 2021;14(4):e000102.
2. Harjola V-P, Mullens W, Banaszewski M, et al. Organ dysfunction, injury and failure in acute heart failure: from pathophysiology to diagnosis and management. A review on behalf of the Acute Heart Failure Committee of the Heart Failure Association (HFA) of the European Society of Cardiology (ESC). Eur J Heart Fail 2017; 19(7):821–36.
3. Nikolaou M, Parissis J, Yilmaz MB, et al. Liver function abnormalities, clinical profile, and outcome in acute decompensated heart failure. Eur Heart J 2013;34(10): 742–9.
4. Hilscher M, Sanchez W. Congestive hepatopathy. Clin Liver Dis 2016;8:68–71. https://doi.org/10.1002/cld.573.
5. El Hadi H, Di Vincenzo A, Vettor R, et al. Relationship between heart disease and Liver disease: a two-way street. Cells 2020;9(3):567.
6. Koehne de Gonzalez AK, Lefkowitch JH. Heart disease and the liver: Pathologic evaluation. Gastroenterol Clin North Am 2017;46(2):421–35.
7. Bosch DE, Koro K, Richards E, et al. Validation of a congestive hepatic fibrosis scoring system. Am J Surg Pathol 2019;43(6):766–72.
8. Fortea JI, Puente Á, Cuadrado A, et al. Congestive hepatopathy. Int J Mol Sci 2020;21(24):9420.
9. Bozkurt B. What is new in heart failure management in 2017? Update on ACC/AHA heart failure guidelines. Curr Cardiol Rep 2018;20(6):39.
10. Ventetuolo CE, Klinger JR. Management of acute right ventricular failure in the intensive care unit. Ann Am Thorac Soc 2014;11(5):811–22.
11. Liang W, He X, Wu D, et al. Prognostic implication of liver function tests in heart failure with preserved ejection fraction without chronic hepatic diseases: Insight from TOPCAT trial. Front Cardiovasc Med 2021;8:618816. https://doi.org/10.3389/fcvm.2021.618816.
12. Thandavarayan RA, Chitturi KR, Guha A. Pathophysiology of acute and chronic right heart failure. Cardiol Clin 2020;38(2):149–60.
13. Arrigo M, Huber LC, Winnik S, et al. Right ventricular failure: pathophysiology, diagnosis and treatment. Card Fail Rev 2019;5(3):140–6.
14. Konstam MA, Kiernan MS, Bernstein D, et al. Evaluation and management of right-sided heart failure: a scientific statement from the American heart association. Circulation 2018;137(20):e578–622.
15. Xanthopoulos A, Starling RC, Kitai T, et al. Heart failure and liver disease: Cardiohepatic interactions. JACC Heart Fail 2019;7(2):87–97.
16. Correale M, Tarantino N, Petrucci R, et al. Liver disease and heart failure: Back and forth. Eur J Intern Med 2018;48:25–34. https://doi.org/10.1016/j.ejim.2017.10.016.

17. Lemmer A, VanWagner L, Ganger D. Congestive hepatopathy: Differentiating congestion from fibrosis. Clin Liver Dis (Hoboken) 2018;10(6):139–43.

18. Biecker E. Diagnosis and therapy of ascites in liver cirrhosis. World J Gastroenterol 2011;17(10):1237–48.

19. Allen LA, Stevenson LW, Grady KL, et al. Decision making in advanced heart failure: a scientific statement from the American Heart Association. Circulation 2012; 125(15):1928–52.

Trends in Reduction of Mortality in Liver Trauma

Whitney Villegas, DNP, AGACNP-BC[a],[1], Jeanette Vaughan, DNP, RN, CCRN, CNL[b],*

KEYWORDS

- Liver trauma • Hepatic injury • Nonoperative management • WSES standards

KEY POINTS

- Management trends in liver trauma changed in 2018 with focus on early computed tomography scanning to determine severity of injury
- Management with multidisciplinary trauma teams
- More focus on nonoperative management to reduce mortality

INTRODUCTION

The paradigm has shifted to reduce mortality in liver trauma. Liver injury remains a leading cause of death in abdominal trauma, mostly resulting from exsanguination.[1–3] However, advancements in multidisciplinary assessment standards, damage control surgery, assertive computed tomography (CT) scans, and management to avoid the lethal triad of acidosis, hypothermia, and coagulopathy have reduced mortality.[1–4] In 2018, the American association for the surgery of trauma (AAST) updated liver grading criteria to incorporate active contrast extravasation and the containment of vascular injury to improve outcomes.[5]

Liver trauma severity is determined with grade. With blunt abdominal trauma, 85% of injury comprised is low grade (grades 1–3) and 15% high grade (grades 4–5).[6] The most common blunt liver injury occurs with motor vehicle collision.[7] Other mechanisms include autopedestrian and falls.[8] In penetrating liver trauma, 40% of abdominal stab wounds and 30% of gunshot wound injure the liver.[7] A major obstacle for the treatment of liver injury are comorbidities of the victim, which increase morbidity.[9]

Clinical Relevance and Diagnostics

Positioned under the right coastal margin, the liver is the largest intra-abdominal organ. It is divided into 2 lobes. The common hepatic artery provides about 25% of

[a] Trauma and Acute Care Emergency Surgery, John Peter Smith Health Network; [b] Louisiana State University Health Sciences Center New Orleans
[1] Present address: 12,256 Indian Creek Drive, Fort Worth, TX 76179.
* Corresponding author. 212 Hollywood Drive, Metairie, LA 70005.
E-mail address: jvaug6@lsuhsc.edu
Twitter: @VaughanJeanette (J.V.)

Crit Care Nurs Clin N Am 34 (2022) 351–359
https://doi.org/10.1016/j.cnc.2022.04.008
0899-5885/22/© 2022 Elsevier Inc. All rights reserved.

blood flow to the liver and a half of its oxygenation. The portal vein provides up to 75% of blood flow and the other half of oxygenation. The hepatic veins are the most damaged structures in the liver, because they are fragile and easily torn.[10]

Blunt trauma to the abdomen is caused by a direct blow causing compression or crushing of the abdomen. Injury is caused by tears or shearing from the force. Shearing injury occurs when there is movement of the mobile liver in relation to the fixed diaphragm.[7] In penetrating trauma, lower energy stab wounds and gunshot wounds cause lacerations and tears. High-energy penetrations cause an increase in damage from blast effects.[7] Liver trauma comprises 5% of all trauma admissions.[8]

On arrival to the emergency department (ED), a full history of the trauma should be obtained to determine the likelihood of liver injury. Details should include location of impact of vehicle, speed of vehicle, and determination of ejection for blunt injuries. For penetrating, the type of weapon, ammunition, and distance between the patient and instrument of injury are important. Use of anticoagulants or history of coagulopathies is also significant.[7] Diagnosis of liver injury can be made using the methods described in **Box 1**. Abdominal examination should include inspection, auscultation, percussion, and palpation.[7] The presence of abrasions, wounds, contusions,

---

Box 1
Diagnostics in liver trauma

Physical Examination Findings
- Vital signs for hemodynamic stability
- Systematic abdominal examination
  - Abrasions, wounds, contusions, abdominal distention[7]
  - Right upper quadrant tenderness (distinguish between light and deep palpation)[7]
  - Involuntary guarding = possible peritonitis[7]
- Bedside exploration of stab wounds to determine depth[3]

Laboratory Studies
- Standard trauma laboratories: CBC, CMP, Coags, lactate[8]
- Serum liver enzymes (AST, ALT) likely elevated[9,13]

Computer Tomography Scan
- Done in hemodynamically stable patients[11,12]
- High accuracy to identify injury and determining the extent of injury (grading)[5,6]
- Done in penetrating injury to determine the stab wound tract or bullet trajectory[3]
- Active bleeding seems as a contrast "blush" (pooling of IV contrast within the liver parenchyma)[12]

Focused Assessment of Sonography for Trauma (FAST)
- Ultrasound used to detect fluid as an indicator of injury[7,11]
- Quick, noninvasive, inexpensive, and can enable triage to the operating room[7,11]
- Signs of liver injury on FAST: subcapsular or perihepatic fluid, fluid in the perihepatic space[6,7,10]
- High specificity, low sensitivity (positive FAST proves the presence of injury but negative FAST does not exclude the possibility of injury)[6,11]
- Should not be used exclusively for diagnosis

Diagnostic peritoneal lavage
- Optional diagnostic tool for unstable patients with suspected abdominal trauma (blunt or penetrating) to determine the need for operation[7,11]
- Catheter is inserted into the peritoneum and fluid is aspirated to assess for blood, bile, or gastrointestinal contents. If no fluid is obtained, then lavage is performed[7]
- Significant false-positive rate[7,11]

distention, right upper quadrant tenderness, or guarding indicates possible injury to the liver.[8] Rapid use of Focused Assessment of Sonography for Trauma (FAST) is part of the initial trauma workup.[11] Suspected injury is confirmed with CT scan as the gold standard.[11,12] CT is highly accurate in determining the extent of injury, active bleeding, vascular compromise, or biliary complications.[2,6] Although diagnostic peritoneal lavage can be done rapidly at bedside, it is invasive and has a significant false-positive rate.[11]

Liver injuries are graded based on the severity of injury (**Table 1**). The Liver Injury Scale by the AAST considers the severity of liver hematoma, laceration, and vascular injury shown on CT scan or in the operating room.[5] The World Society of Emergency Surgery (WSES) has also developed a scale to supplement the AAST scoring system, which includes hemodynamic status.[3] Following initial trauma evaluation to determine the grade of injury, assessment of hemodynamic status, identification of other injuries, and medical comorbidities will help make the decision on whether to pursue imminent surgery or nonoperative treatment.[7]

NONOPERATIVE TREATMENT

Nonoperative treatment has become the treatment of choice for patients with liver trauma who are hemodynamically stable, even in high-grade injuries.[3,12,14] Nonoperative treatment has shown to reduce mortality, hospital costs, length of stay, blood transfusions, and abdominal complications.[6,10,12,14] Patients with penetrating liver injuries can be managed nonoperatively if the wound does not enter the peritoneum.[3] Treatment consists of monitoring with serial hemoglobin level and abdominal examinations.[3,12] The patient is usually kept NPO and on bedrest during the early phases of monitoring and may be monitored in the ICU for the first several days.[8,9,12] Current

Table 1
Liver injury grades

AAST Grade[5]	Criteria[5]	WSES Grade with Hemodynamic Stability[3]
I	• Subcapsular hematoma surface area: <10% • Parenchymal laceration depth: <1 cm • Capsular tear	I (Minor) Stable
II	• Subcapsular hematoma surface area: 10%–50% • Intraparenchymal hematoma <10 cm diameter • Laceration depth: 1–3 cm • Laceration length: ≤10 cm	I (Minor) Stable
III	• Subcapsular hematoma surface area: >50% • Ruptured hematoma (subcapsular or parenchymal) • Intraparenchymal hematoma >10 cm • Laceration depth: >3 cm • Liver vascular injury or active bleeding contained in the liver parenchyma	II (Moderate) Stable
IV	• Parenchymal disruption of 25%–75% of a lobe • Active bleeding extending beyond the parenchyma into peritoneum	III (Severe) Stable
V	• Parenchymal disruption >75 of a lobe • Venous injuries including vena cava and major hepatic veins	III (Severe) Stable
		IV (Severe) Any AAST grade, unstable

guidelines for liver trauma do not have recommendations for the optimal timing to resume diet, activity, or anticoagulants to prevent venous thromboembolism, so practices vary among facilities.[12] Generally, a patient can resume normal activities 3 to 4 months after injury if no complications occur.[3]

Nonoperative treatment fails in up to one-third of patients due to bleeding, missed injuries of the gastrointestinal tract, or abdominal compartment syndrome.[6] Patients with high-grade liver injuries, additional traumatic injuries, and lower Glasgow Coma Scale are at a higher risk for failure.[14] Angioembolization is often used in nonoperative liver trauma patients who have concerns for active bleeding and has a 93% success rate in stopping arterial hemorrhage.[15] For angioembolization, the patient is taken to the interventional radiology suite, where angiography is performed and coils, glue, or gelfoam is used to stop active bleeding or prevent further bleeding.[16] Although angioembolization has relatively low complication rates, these patients are at an increased risk of hepatic necrosis due to decreased blood flow to the liver.[6]

OPERATIVE MANAGEMENT

Patients who are unstable in the ED despite initial fluid resuscitation should be taken to the operating room.[3,12] This has been defined as systolic blood pressure less than 90, heart rate greater then 120, evidence of vasoconstriction/shock (such as cool clammy skin and decreased capillary refill), altered level of consciousness, and shortness of breath.[12] Up to 35% of complex (high-grade) liver injuries will require operation, either initially or due to failed nonoperative treatment.[14] Ninety percent of high-energy penetrating liver injuries requires surgery.[3] Many patients with liver trauma require surgery for other abdominal injuries, such as of the bowel or spleen.[12]

Surgery on the liver for traumatic injury requires complex techniques.[13] Patients with life-threatening bleeding undergo damage control surgery, which focuses on hemorrhage control and control of gastrointestinal contamination of the abdomen.[8,10,13] At the same time, the patient is resuscitated to achieve hemostasis; blood products should be given in a 1:1:1 ratio of packed red blood cells to fresh frozen plasma to platelets.[10] During damage control surgery, the abdomen is often packed and temporarily closed to allow for further resuscitation with correction of acidosis, coagulopathy, and hypothermia in the intensive care unit.[13] Leaving the abdominal skin and fascia open during the resuscitation period helps reduce the risk of abdominal compartment syndrome, although it can still occur in patients with an open abdomen.[10] The patient will then return to the OR in 24 to 48 hours for the removal of packing and further intervention.[10,13] The longer packs are left in place, the higher the risk of sepsis.[10]

During surgery for liver trauma, bleeding may be controlled by compression, packing, cautery, topical hemostatic agents and other coagulation methods, ligation of blood vessels, and balloon tamponade.[3,8,14] The parenchyma of the liver can be directly repaired with sutures (called hepatorrhaphy), and damage to large vessels and bile ducts may also be repaired.[8] Liver tissue may require debridement or resection if necrosis is present.[14] After surgery, drains may be left in place to control bile leaks or hepatic necrosis.[8] Angio-embolization can be performed in addition to surgery (either in the operating room or postoperatively) to help control bleeding.[3,10]

Liver transplant for trauma has been successfully performed but is extremely rare.[10,17] A patient could qualify for transplant if they fail or cannot undergo typical treatment, develop extensive hepatic necrosis, or have progressive liver failure from their injury.[10] However, the patient must also have minimal other traumatic injuries, be stable enough to survive the transplant surgery, and have a donor organ immediately available.[10]

COMPLICATIONS

Patients with traumatic liver injury are at risk of numerous complications, some of which are outlined in **Table 2**. Complications following hepatic injury are reported in 11% to 16% of patients and increase with liver injury grade.[2] Nonoperative complications include bleeding, bile leak, hepatic necrosis, abscess, fistulas, thrombosis, and pseudoaneurysm of hepatic vasculature.[14] Biliary complications are the most common and are typically found later in the hospital course.[3,12] Complications may lead to additional procedures and longer hospital stays.

NURSING CONSIDERATIONS

The primary nursing consideration after ensuring adequate airway and oxygenation for a patient with liver trauma is hemodynamic stability.[19] Frequent vital signs and physical assessments for complications should be completed. Intravenous access should include 2 large bore catheters to sustain fluid resuscitation. Controlling the patient's pain without sedation is the next task. This is generally accomplished with opioids.[20]

Care of the liver trauma patient in the ICU is multifaceted. Serial blood draws including hemoglobin and hematocrits, complete blood counts, coagulopathy indicators (such as partial prothrombin times and international normalized ratio), platelet counts, lactate, and liver enzymes. These values will help predict complications such as hemorrhagic shock, sepsis, liver failure, and organ dysfunction.[19] Vasopressors should not be used in the early stages of trauma because stabilization with fluids improves microcirculation and oxygen balance of vital organs.[19,21]

Because many liver trauma patients sustain polytrauma, they may be intubated and mechanically ventilated. Intubation prolongs ICU length of stay and may predispose patients to hospital acquired infections and increased mortality.[22] Weaning from mechanical ventilation via protocols should begin early to prevent complications. Nasogastric tube insertion will keep the patient's stomach decompressed and prevent aspiration.[20] Urine output should be monitored to assess for hypoperfusion. With penetrating liver trauma, tetanus prophylaxis should be initiated.

The nursing physical assessment is important for monitoring in both operative and nonoperative liver trauma. Inspection for seat belt ecchymosis should be noted. Bruising around the flank (Grey-Turner sign) could signal retro-peritoneal hemorrhage but may not show for hours after the trauma.[20] Auscultation should include notation of abdominal bruits, which could indicate hepatic vascular injury.[23] If right upper quadrant pain is severe, nursing assessment with percussion and palpation should be deferred.[20] An increase in abdominal rigidity, a sudden increase in pain, or decrease in hemoglobin and hematocrit could indicate hemorrhage. Hypothermia or changes to serial laboratory values, including lactate, H and H, and arterial blood gases should be noted. The trauma team should be notified urgently for any changes in condition because they may point to complications.[24,25]

Patients who sustain major trauma require long-term recovery and rehabilitation. A significant number of patients experience mental health issues, including social dysfunction, depression, anxiety, and posttraumatic stress disorder.[26] Nurses should be attuned to altered coping mechanisms that could ultimately affect recovery, and victims of violence should be referred to victim support groups.[24] Victims may fear retaliation after trauma, especially if the liver trauma sustained was due to gunfire or stabbings.

Key members of the interdisciplinary team include social workers to address long-term recovery efforts and mental health professionals.[26] Often families are stunned after someone sustains life-threatening trauma. They may or may not have been aware of the patient's life choices making it difficult to cope. Chaplains should also be

Table 2
Complications of liver trauma

Complication	Definition/Patho	Liver Injury Population	Symptoms/Presentation	Treatment
Bile leak	• From injury or necrosis to the bile ducts • Can cause irritation and inflammation of the peritoneum (bile peritonitis)[16]	• Operative (majority) • Nonoperative • Postembolization[15,18]	• Elevated bilirubin • Abdominal distention • Food intolerance • Possible sepsis[10,18]	• Various, including percutaneous drain, ERCP, or operative[12]
Hemobilia	• Bleeding from and into the biliary tract from fistula formation[10]	• Blunt trauma • Nonoperative • Operative	• Right upper quadrant pain • Jaundice • Upper GI bleeding • Decreasing hemoglobin[10]	• Angioembolization
Rebleeding or delayed hemorrhage	• Usually occurs due to ruptured subcapsular hematoma or pseudoaneurysm[3]	• Nonoperative	• Hemodynamic instability • Decreasing Hemoglobin	• Embolization, nonoperative, or operative[3]
Liver abscess	• From contamination from bile ducts or vasculature; or from hepatic necrosis[15]	• Postembolization • Operative • Uncommonly nonoperative[15]	• Signs of sepsis • Abnormal LFTs • Abdominal pain • Food intolerance[10]	• Antibiotics, • Percutaneous drain placement[3]
Hepatic necrosis	• Necrosis of liver from disruption of blood flow, which can lead to further complications, such as bile leaks, clotting problems, respiratory compromise, sepsis[3,10,12]	• Postembolization • Operative	• Elevated AST/ALT • Bleeding • Abdominal pain • Food intolerance • Signs of sepsis[10]	• Operative debridement or resection[3]
Abdominal compartment syndrome	• Increased intra-abdominal pressure resulting in decreased blood flow and organ dysfunction[10]	• Nonoperative • Operative	• Elevated bladder pressure • Abdominal distention • Decreased urine output	• Decompressive laparotomy[10]

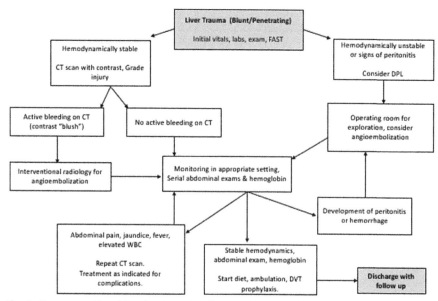

Fig. 1. Treatment Algorithm for traumatic liver injury.

available for consult. In poor outcomes postliver trauma, where demise is imminent, nurses should consider consultation of organ procurement services.

CASE STUDY

A 92 year-old woman was admitted to the trauma ICU following surgical intervention for a grade IV liver laceration due to motor vehicle collision. The patient was the driver and sustained a T-bone blunt impact from the other vehicle at 50 mph. Initial trauma evaluation included FAST and revealed hemorrhage into the abdomen, which CT confirmed. Due to hemodynamic instability, she was taken to the OR where liver resection took place for more than 3.5 hours. On arrival to the ICU, she was intubated and ventilated. Initially, she was hemodynamically stable; however, 35 minutes after arrival, she began having coupled PVCs followed by a short run of V-tach. This was followed by cardiac arrest due to ventricular tachycardia. On arrival of the crash cart, she was defibrillated a total of 5 times during ACLS resuscitation. In evaluation of the 6 Hs and 5 Ts, her POC glucose was 103, BP before arrest was 132/79, HR was 93, RR on the ventilator was 22, and she was assisting. Oxygen saturations were 95% on a PEEP of 5 cm, FiO_2 35%. Arterial blood gases during the code were pH of 7.34, HCO_3 28, PO_2 63, and CO_2 37. Bagging revealed no obstruction. End tidal CO_2 was 44. Attending surgeon, nurses, and resuscitation team continued to review the 6 Hs. Several rounds of epinephrine and 2 rounds of amiodarone had been given, yet the V-tach persisted. Finally, the bedside nurse asked, "Has anyone gotten a recent temperature?" That assessment had been missed during initial receipt of patient from the OR. On obtaining a temperature, it was found to be hypothermic at 93.8 F. Normal saline for resuscitation was transferred immediately to a blood warmer and infused rapidly. After several minutes of thermoregulatory therapy, her rectal temperature improved. She was again defibrillated, this time with success. She converted to a slow sinus rhythm. Lesson learned? Do not forget the all-important temperature as a part of initial assessment **Fig. 1.**

CLINICS CARE POINTS

Evidence-based-nursing implications include the following:

- Maintaining hemodynamic stability
- Monitoring for signs and symptoms of hemorrhage
- Pain management
- Assessment of laboratories including H/H and coags
- Addressing psychosocial and emotional issues of trauma

DISCLOSURE

The authors have nothing to disclose.

REFERENCES

1. Tagkalos E, Jöckel M, Lang H, et al. Treatment of blunt liver injuries after the paradigm shift in liver trauma management. HPB (Oxford, England) 2019;21:S794.
2. Wagner ML, Streit S, Makley AT, et al. Hepatic pseudoaneurysm incidence after liver trauma. J Surg Res 2020;256:623–8.
3. Coccolini F, Catena F, Moore EE, et al. WSES classification and guidelines for liver trauma. World J Emerg Surg 2016;11:50.
4. Suen K, Skandarajah AR, Knowles B, et al. Changes in the management of liver trauma leading to reduced mortality: 15-year experience in a major trauma centre: changes in management of liver trauma. ANZ J Surg 2016;86:894–9.
5. Kozar RA, Crandall M, Shanmuganathan K, et al. Organ injury scaling 2018 update: spleen, liver, and kidney. J Trauma acute Care Surg 2018;85:1119.
6. Roberts R, Sheth RA. Hepatic trauma. Ann translational Med 2021;9:1195.
7. American College of Surgeons Committee on Trauma. ATLS™ advanced trauma life support Student course Manual. 10th edition. American College of Surgeons; 2018.
8. Taghavi S, Askari R. Liver trauma. StatPearls. Updated July; 2021. Available at: https://www.ncbi.nlm.nih.gov/books/NBK513236/. Accessed December 1, 2021.
9. Kaptanoglu L, Kurt N, Sikar HE. Current approach to liver Traumas. Int J Surg (London, England) 2017;39:255–9.
10. Bruns BR, Kozar RA. Liver and biliary tract. In: Moore EE, Feliciano DV, Mattox KL, editors. Trauma. 8th edition. McGraw Hill; 2017. p. 551–73.
11. Stengel D, Rademacher G, Ekkernkamp A, et al. Emergency ultrasound-based algorithms for diagnosing blunt abdominal trauma. Cochrane Libr 2015;2015: CD004446.
12. Stassen NA, Bhullar I, Cheng JD, et al. Nonoperative management of blunt hepatic injury: an Eastern Association for the Surgery of Trauma practice management guideline. J Trauma acute Care Surg 2012;73:S288.
13. Doklestic K, Loncar Z, Bumbasirevic V, et al. Surgical management of AAST grades III-V hepatic trauma by Damage control surgery with perihepatic packing and Definitive hepatic repair-single centre experience. World J Emerg Surg 2015;10:34.
14. Ingraham A, Peitzman AB. Abdominal trauma. In: Vincent J-L, Abraham E, Moore FA, et al, editors. Textbook of Critical care. 7th edition. Elsevier; 2017. p. 1188–90.

15. Green CS, Bulger EM, Kwan SW. Outcomes and complications of angioemboliza-
    tion for hepatic trauma: a systematic review of the literature. J Trauma acute Care
    Surg 2016;80:529.
16. Gilyard S, Shinn K, Nezami N, et al. Contemporary management of hepatic
    trauma: what IRs need to Know. Semin Interv Radiol 2020;37:035–43.
17. Riberio MAF, Medrado MB, Rosa M, et al. Liver transplantation after severe hepat-
    ic trauma: Current indications and results. Arquivos Brasileiros de cirurgia diges-
    tiva: ABCD. 2015;28:28 286–289.
18. Virdis F, Reccia I, Di Saverio S, et al. Clinical outcomes of primary arterial embo-
    lization in severe hepatic trauma: a systematic review. Diagn Interv Imaging 2019;
    100:65–75.
19. Andrei S, Isac S, Carstea M, et al. Isolated liver trauma: a clinical perspective in a
    non-emergency center for liver surgery. Exp Ther Med 2021;2022–3.
20. Blank-Reid C. Abdominal trauma. Nursing 2007;37:4–11. https://doi.org/10.1097/
    01.NURSE.0000266090.38090.76.
21. Gupta B, Garg N, Ramachandran R. Vasopressors: do they have any role in hem-
    orrhagic shock? J anaesthesiololgy Clin Pharmacol 2017;33:3–8.
22. Okabe Y. Risk factors for prolonged mechanical ventilation in patients with severe
    multiple injuries and blunt chest trauma: a single center retrospective case-
    control study. Acute Med Surg 2018;5:166–72.
23. Lada NE, Gupta A, Anderson SW, et al. Liver trauma: hepatic vascular injury on
    computed tomography as a predictor of patient outcome. Eur Radiol 2020;31:
    3375–82.
24. Emergency Nurses Association. TNCC provider Manual. 8th edition. Jones and
    Bartlett; 2020.
25. Edwards M, Laing R. 226 management of liver trauma: outcomes at one of Eu-
    rope's most active HPB and liver transplant Centres. Br J Surg 2021;108.
26. Herrera-Escobar JP, Rivero R, Apoj M, et al. Long-term social dysfunction after
    trauma: what is the prevalence, risk factors, and associated outcomes? Surgery
    2019;166:392–7.

Moving?

Make sure your subscription moves with you!

To notify us of your new address, find your **Clinics Account Number** (located on your mailing label above your name), and contact customer service at:

Email: journalscustomerservice-usa@elsevier.com

800-654-2452 (subscribers in the U.S. & Canada)
314-447-8871 (subscribers outside of the U.S. & Canada)

Fax number: 314-447-8029

Elsevier Health Sciences Division
Subscription Customer Service
3251 Riverport Lane
Maryland Heights, MO 63043

*To ensure uninterrupted delivery of your subscription, please notify us at least 4 weeks in advance of move.

Printed and bound by CPI Group (UK) Ltd, Croydon, CR0 4YY

03/10/2024

01040471-0011